Q&A Color Review of

Hepatobiliary Medicine

Henry C. Bodenheimer, Jr. MD
Beth Israel Medical Center
and
Albert Einstein College of Medicine
New York, USA

Roger Chapman BSc, MD, FRCP
The Oxford Radcliffe Hospital
Oxford, UK

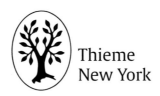

Thieme
New York

Preface

This book is written for gastroenterologists, hepatologists, nurses, medical students, and all health-care providers who treat or care for those with hepatobiliary diseases. The clinical subjects covered are diverse and span both adult and pediatric illnesses. The text features a question and answer format designed to engage the reader. Concise text delivers the most clinically relevant information, guiding up-to-date management of liver and biliary tract disease. The plentiful use of illustrations and the presentation of laboratory data simulates the clinical setting and encourages the reader to test themselves by formulating a diagnosis and management strategy and then learn from the answers provided on the page following.

The topics included in this book were selected to represent the wide spectrum of clinical issues facing a practitioner. In addition to the common problems of viral hepatitis, alcoholic liver disease, and gallstones, we have included information on metabolic disorders, transplantation, cancer, and autoimmune disorders, such as primary sclerosing cholangitis and primary biliary cirrhosis.

We are confident that the reader will find this broad educational experience both informative and fun.

Henry C. Bodenheimer, Jr.
Roger Chapman

First published in the United States of America in 2003 by:
Thieme New York, 333 Seventh Avenue
New York, NY 10001, USA

ISBN 1–58890–152–1

Library of Congress Cataloging-in-Publication Data
is available from the publisher

Important note: Medical knowledge is ever-changing. As new research and clinical experience broaden our knowledge, changes in treatment and drug therapy may be required. The authors and editors of the material herein have consulted sources believed to be reliable in their efforts to provide information that is complete and in accord with the standards accepted at the time of publication. However, in view of the possibility of human error by the authors, editors, or publisher of the work herein, or changes in medical knowledge, neither the authors, editors, or publisher, nor any other party who has been involved in the preparation of this work, warrants that the information contained herein is in every respect accurate or complete, and they are not responsible for any errors or omissions or for the results obtained from use of such information. Readers are encouraged to confirm the information contained herein with other sources. For example, readers are advised to check the product information sheet included in the package of each drug they plan to administer to be certain that the information contained in this publication is accurate and that changes have not been made in the recommended dose or in the contraindications for administration. This recommendation is of particular importance in connection with new or infrequently used drugs.

Some of the product names, patents, and registered designs referred to in this book are in fact registered trademarks or proprietary names even though specific reference to this fact is not always made in the text. Therefore, the appearance of a name without designation as proprietary is not to be construed as a representation by the publisher that it is in the public domain.

Copyright © 2003 Manson Publishing Ltd, 73 Corringham Road, London NW11 7DL, UK

Printed in Spain

Contributors

Imtiaz Alam, BMSc, MBChB
Central Texas Gastroenterology
Round Rock, Texas, USA

Bruce R. Bacon, MD
Saint Louis University School of Medicine
Saint Louis, Missouri, USA

Nathan M. Bass, MB, CHB
University of California
San Francisco, California, USA

Nora V. Bergasa, MD, FACP
Columbia University College of Medicine
New York, New York, USA

Henry C. Bodenheimer, Jr., MD
Beth Israel Medical Center and
Albert Einstein College of Medicine
New York, New York, USA

Ulrika Broomé, MD, PhD
Huddinge University Hospital
Huddinge, Sweden

Roger Chapman, BSc, MD, FRCP
The Oxford Radcliffe Hospital
Oxford, UK

Massimo Colombo, MD
IRCCS Maggiore Hospital University of Milan
Milan, Italy

Linda D. Ferrell, MD
University of California
San Francisco, California, USA

Thomas M. Fishbein, MD
Mount Sinai Medical Center
New York, New York, USA

A. Sánchez Fueyo, MD
Hospital Clínic Provincial
University of Barcelona
Barcelona, Spain

Norman D. Grace, MD
Brigham & Women's Hospital
Boston, Massachusetts, USA

Philip J. Johnson, MD, FRCP
University of Birmingham
Edgbaston, Birmingham, UK

Emmet B. Keeffe, MD
Stanford University Medical Center
Palo Alto, California, USA

Eduardo A. Kofman, MD
Brownsville Medical Center
Brownsville, Texas, USA

Charles S. Lieber, MD, MACP
Veterans Affairs Medical Center
Bronx, New York, USA

John Martin, MA, MRCP
Chelsea and Westminster Hospital
London, UK

Charles M. Miller, MD
Mount Sinai Medical Center
New York, New York, USA

Kelvin R. Palmer, MD, FRCP (Ed.),
FRCP (Lond.)
Western General Hospital NHS Trust
Edinburgh, UK

Andrew Pascoe, MD
The Oxford Radcliffe Hospital
Oxford, UK

J. Rodés, MD
Hospital Clínic Provincial
University of Barcelona
Barcelona, Spain

Philip Rosenthal, MD
University of California
San Francisco, California, USA

Floriano Rosina, MD
Azienda Ospedaliera San Giovanni Battista di
Torino
Torino, Italy

Alberto Sanchez-Fueyo, MD
Hospital Clinic
Barcelona, Spain

Michael L. Schilsky, MD
Mount Sinai Medical Center
New York, New York, USA

Samuel H. Sigal, MD
Mount Sinai Medical Center
New York, New York, USA

Max W. Sung, MD
Mount Sinai Medical Center
New York, New York, USA

Kate Tonge, MRCP
Hillingdon Hospital
Uxbridge, UK

Normal ranges

Albumin (serum) 3.7–4.78 mg/dL (2.59–5.18 mmol/L)
Alkaline phosphatase (ALP) 37–116 U/L
Alphafetoprotein (serum) 0–20 ng/mL
Alanine aminotransferase (ALT) (SGPT) 5–40 U/L
Aspartate aminotransferase (AST) (SGOT) 5–40 U/L
Bicarbonate 18–23 mEq/L (18–23 mmol/L)
Bilirubin
    direct-reacting 0–0.2 mg/dL (0–3.4 µmol/L)
    total 0.1–1 mg/dL (1.7–17.1 µmol/L)
Blood urea nitrogen (BUN) 7–25 mg/dL
Ceruloplasmin 20–40 mg/dL (200–400 mg/L)
Chloride 98–106 mEq/L (98–106 mmol/L)
Cholesterol 100–200 mg/dL (2.6–5.2 mmol/L)
Creatinine <1.5 mg/dL (<133 µmol/L)
Erythrocyte sedimentation rate (ESR) 1–20 mm/hour
Estrogen 4.0–11.6 ng/dL
Ferritin 14–200 µg/L
Gammaglobulin 0.6 g/dL (6–16 g/L)
Gamma-glutamytranspeptidase (GGTP) 10–46 U/L
Glucose 75–115 mg/dL (4.2–6.4 mmol/L)
Hematocrit 38.5–45.0%
Hemoglobin 11.2–15.6 g/dL (112–156 g/L)
Immunoglobulin M (IgM) 50–320 mg/dL (0.5–3.2 g/L)
Internal normalized ratio (INR) 0.9–1.1
Iron 35–175 µg/dL
Leukocytes 4,000–11,000/mm^3 (4.0–11.0 $\times$ 10^9/L)
Luteinizing hormone 2–12 U/L
Mean cell volume (MCV) 75–96 fl
Partial thromboplastin time 25–38 seconds
Platelet count 150–400,000/mm^3 (150–400 $\times$ 10^9/L)
Potassium 3.5–5.0 mEq/L (3.5–5.0 mmol/L)
Prothrombin time 12 seconds
Sodium 135–145 mEq/L (135–145 mmol/L)
Testosterone 225–900 ng/dL (78–312 nmol/L)
Total iron binding capacity (TIBC) 45–75 µmol/L
Transferrin saturation 15–50%
Triglycerides <160 mg/dL (<1.8 mmol/L)
White blood cell (WBC) 3,000–10,000/mm^3 (3–10 $\times$ 10^9/L)

1 A 62-year-old male has been in the intensive care unit for 3 weeks with sepsis and adult respiratory distress syndrome. Fever and leukocytosis present on admission have resolved with the use of broad spectrum antibiotics, but he has developed a persistent ileus.

AST 80 U/L
ALT 60 U/L
Albumin 2.8 g/dL (28 g/L)
Bilirubin 1.0 mg/dl (17.1 μmol/l)
ALP 100 U/L
Prothrombin time 12.2 seconds

He has been receiving TPN at a rate of 3 L/day for 8 days. The dextrose concentration of the TPN has been maintained at 25%; no intravenous fat emulsion has been included. The changes in biochemical liver tests are shown.

The patient had been on multiple medications, which had been discontinued 3 days before starting TPN. Physical examination revealed a weight of 110 lb (50 kg) and an enlarged liver with a span of 13 cm (5 in). An abdominal CT scan is performed and reveals a low attenuation of the liver relative to the spleen.

i. What is the likely etiology of the changes in the biochemical liver tests?

ii. What factors contribute to the development of this condition?

iii. What are the two most important initial steps in the management of this patient?

iv. What treatment should be considered if hepatic enzymes continue to increase?

2 Are CT scans and, or, MRI of the liver useful tests in the evaluation of iron overload?

What features of the CT (**2a**) and MRI (**2b**) scans may indicate increased hepatic iron content?

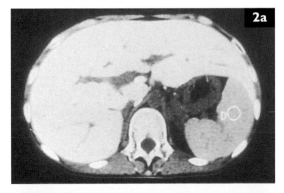

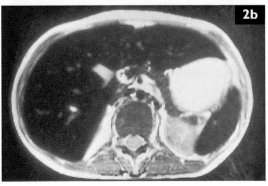

1 i. The patient has probably developed mild hepatic steatosis secondary to TPN. A variety of abnormalities in liver tests may also be associated with systemic infection but these typically include hyperbilirubinemia and increased serum ALP. Also, the sepsis was controlled at the advent of the biochemical liver test abnormalities. The low albumin may reflect decreased production as an acute phase reaction to illness. Finally, the CT findings are strongly suggestive of fatty infiltration of the liver.

ii. Factors contributing to the development of steatosis are excessive carbohydrate calorie administration via TPN and a lack of lipid infusion. Calories should be delivered at a rate of 25–30 kcal/kg bodyweight, as a balanced mixture of carbo-hydrates and fat. Hypercaloric TPN, especially with excess dextrose, can promote and worsen hepatic steatosis. A lipid emulsion comprising no more than one third of the total calorie intake should be simultaneously infused during TPN therapy to reduce and sometimes reverse the development of hepatic steatosis.

iii. The initial steps in the management of this patient would be to confirm that all potentially hepatotoxic medications have been discontinued, and to ensure that TPN is appropriately balanced in terms of carbohydrate calories, fat calories, and total calorie requirements.

iv. Efforts to initiate enteral feeding should begin as soon as possible. Other steps, including cyclic TPN, minimizing exposure of TPN solutions to light to avoid photo-decomposition, administration of metronidazole or the administration of the amino acid taurine, have also been advocated as potentially useful.

Hepatobiliary abnormalities caused by TPN in adults are diverse in pathophysiology, generally reversible, and usually less severe than those seen in infants. Steatosis, steatohepatitis, and intrahepatic cholestasis occur relatively early in therapy (5–28 days),whereas steatonecrosis, fibrosis, and cirrhosis usually develop only in patients receiving long term TPN (longer than 6 months). TPN induced hepatic steatosis in adults may be the result of decreased fatty acid oxidation, increased fatty acid synthesis, or increased influx of fatty acid synthesis. Decreased lipoprotein synthesis and secretion may also contribute. Allowing for a carbohydrate-free period by intermittently discontinuing or cycling TPN reduces serum glucose concentrations and avoids long periods of elevated insulin levels that may stimulate hepatic fatty acid synthesis.

2 CT scanning and MRI have been proposed for adjunctive use in diagnosing hemochromatosis. The CT from a patient with severe iron overload (**2a**) shows the density of the liver is equivalent to that of bone (vertebral body) and greater than that of the spleen. CT scanning makes the liver light or white. An MRI image (**2b**) from a patient with severe iron overload shows a dark or black liver. The advantage of using these imaging modalities as diagnostic tools is that they are noninvasive. The dis-advantages are that neither method can provide reliable hepatic iron quantification for subsequent calculation of hepatic iron index. There is also no ability to assess for tissue damage such as fibrosis or cirrhosis. These imaging modalities should not replace the use of liver biopsy to definitively establish a diagnosis of hereditary hemo-chromatosis, particularly in patients with suspected liver injury.

3 A 75-year-old female presents with fever, jaundice, and abdominal pain.

i. What test should be urgently performed?

ii. What abnormalities are shown (3)?

iii. How should the patient be managed?

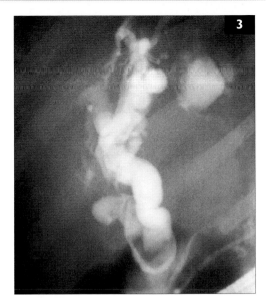

4 A 39-year-old Chinese businessman travelling to Europe presents with fatigue, anorexia, jaundice, and elevated ALT. He denies risk factors for viral hepatitis or heavy alcohol consumption. On admission, the liver is tender with a 14 cm (5.5 in) span. The spleen is palpable. Laboratory investigations are shown.

i. What is the diagnosis?

ii. What is the epidemiology and natural history of this disease?

ALT 1,740 U/L
AST 1,680 U/L
Bilirubin 11 mg/dL (188 μmol/L)
ALP twice upper normal limits
HBsAg absent
Anti-HBs present
Anti-HBc present
Total anti-HAV present
IgM anti-HAV absent
IgM anti-HEV present

5 Which of the following is true of autoimmune hepatitis?

A A positive diagnosis cannot be made, nor should treatment be initiated until signs and, or, symptoms have been present for more than 6 months, i.e. until chronicity has been confirmed.

B The target antigen for the autoimmune reaction is unknown.

C More than 90% of patients have the HLA A1, B8, DR3 haplotype.

D The condition is part of the spectrum of systemic lupus erythematosus.

E Patients have a no higher incidence of other autoimmune diseases than the normal population.

F None of the above.

3 i. Endoscopic retrograde cholangiopancreatography (ERCP). In this examination a duodenoscope is passed into the second part of the duodenum and a cannula is introduced into the biliary and pancreatic ducts. Radiological contrast material is then injected to opacify both the biliary and pancreatic systems.

ii. A large common bile duct calculus and an intrahepatic collection, which is almost certainly an abscess.

iii. With intravenous fluids and intravenous antibiotics. The antibiotic of choice is probably ciprofloxacin. Piperacillin or a combination of a cephalosporin and gentamycin are alternatives. Coagulation defects should be corrected. Following cholangiography the bile duct should be drained and cleared of calculi by first performing a biliary sphincterotomy. This facilitates extraction of common bile duct stones using baskets or balloons. This case involves a very large common bile duct calculus, and stones >2 cm (>0.8 in) in diameter are often too big to be removed. Stones can be crushed using mechanical lithotripsy. If it is not possible to remove the stone, it is wise to leave a plastic stent across the stone enabling infected bile to drain. In this case it is very likely that the hepatic abscess communicates with the biliary tree and is a complication of the gallstone. Percutaneous drainage of the abscess is probably unnecessary but should be considered if the cavity persists on ultrasound examination or if there is evidence of continuing sepsis.

4 i. Acute infection with hepatitis E virus. This is an enterically transmitted, nonenveloped RNA virus which belongs to the family of caliciviruses.

ii. Hepatitis E virus is a major cause of sporadic and epidemic hepatitis in developing countries. Epidemics have been reported in New Dehli, Kanpur, and Xingiang affecting hundreds of thousands of people who drank contaminated water. Sporadic cases have been reported worldwide, including in western countries. Hepatitis E virus causes a self-limited cholestatic form of hepatitis, with an incubation period of 15–64 days. Disease presents with jaundice during outbreaks; mild or subclinical forms are common in sporadic cases. Subacute hepatic failure or late onset fulminant hepatitis cases have been reported to occur in many parts of India. There is no evidence of chronic sequelae and fatal cases were recorded mainly among pregnant women. Standard immune globulin does not protect against hepatitis E virus and a vaccine is not available.

5 None is true. In the past it was difficult to distinguish between acute and chronic active hepatitis; hence the requirement for a confirmed history of over 6 months. However, now good serology can accurately diagnose acute viral hepatitis. Using the high titers of autoantibodies, a confident diagnosis of autoimmune hepatitis can now usually be made without waiting for 6 months. A major target antigen, the asialoglycoprotein receptor, has been identified in autoimmune hepatitis. The haplotype A1, B8, DR3 is more common in autoimmune hepatitis but still only occurs in about 30% of cases. Autoimmune hepatitis is not part of the spectrum of systemic lupus erythematosus although the autoantibody profile is similar. Autoimmune hepatitis patients have a significantly higher rate of other autoimmune diseases, particularly thyroditis and autoimmune hemolysis, than the normal population.

6 A 32-year-old Caucasian female is 31 weeks pregnant and presents with a 1 month history of generalized itch and dark urine. There is no history of fever or abdominal pain. Her first pregnancy 10 years ago was also associated with itching. There is no family history of liver

Bilirubin 3.3 mg/dL (56 µmol/L)
ALP 450 U/L
AST 120 U/L
GGT normal
Albumin 3.1 g/dL (31 g/L)

disease. She takes no medication. Examination reveals a well appearing woman in late pregnancy with jaundice, palmar erythema, spider angiomata, scratch marks, a non-tender gravid abdomen, and mild ankle edema. Her blood pressure is 110/60 mmHg (14.7/8.0 kPa). Urine dip stick tests are positive for urobilinogen and protein. Laboratory investigations are shown. Her CBC is normal. A right upper quadrant ultrasound scan is normal.

i. What condition has complicated this pregnancy?

ii. Is a liver biopsy indicated?

iii. What treatment would you recommend?

iv. Would you recommend early delivery and are there any special precautions which may relate to this condition?

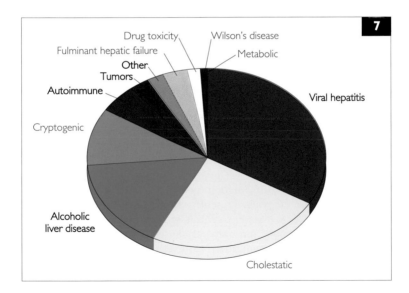

7 The relative contributions of different indications for liver transplantation are shown (7). Which of the disease categories listed below has the highest recurrence rate and poorest outcome after transplant?

A Viral hepatitis.

B Cholestatic disorders.

C Biliary atresia.

D Inherited metabolic disorders.

6 i. In the absence of any underlying liver disease, intrahepatic cholestasis of pregnancy is the likely diagnosis because of itch and jaundice in the third trimester. Pregnant women typically have palmar erythema and spider angiomata which usually disappear postpartum. The low serum albumin is normal for the third trimester of pregnancy. The absence of signs and symptoms of pre-eclampsia and a normal CBC makes HELLP unlikely. Itch is very rare in acute fatty liver of pregnancy which in the majority of patients is characterized by the onset of symptoms at 36 weeks gestation, right upper quadrant/epigastric abnormal pain, a small liver on ultrasound, and hepatic synthetic dysfunction. Bile acids are typically elevated in cholestasis of pregnancy, but not routinely measured. Cholestasis of pregnancy is a syndrome of intrahepatic cholestasis (like primary biliary cirrhosis and drug induced cholestasis), but it occurs in otherwise healthy women in pregnancy or whilst taking oral contraceptives (usually ethinyloestradiol based) and then resolves with no sequelae. Cholestasis of pregnancy is often familial and follows an autosomal dominant pattern of inheritance. Prevalence figures of 1:750–1:7,000 pregnancies have been reported and are probably an underestimate.
ii. Liver biopsy is indicated only very rarely, because the clinical and laboratory findings almost invariably secure the diagnosis. Histology shows intraheptic cholestasis with only minor nonspecific inflammation.
iii. Itch in cholestasis of pregnancy (pruritus gravidarum) typically affects the trunk, extremities (palms and soles), and is worse at night. Both itch and jaundice persist until delivery then resolve rapidly. The only certain remedy for itch relief is delivery but this is generally not needed, cholestasis being a benign affliction for the mother. Cholestyramine is useful for relieving itch and is safe to use. Oral ursodeoxycholic acid 10–15 mg/kg/day is increasingly used in severely affected women. It improves symptoms and biochemistry. Controlled trials are in progress to assess the effect on the fetus.
iv. Prolonged cholestasis of pregnancy may lead to vitamin K deficiency and a prolonged prothrombin time. Parenteral vitamin K should be given before delivery to avoid excessive postpartum bleeding. As intraheptic cholestasis carries an increased risk of fetal dysfunction/prematurity and stillbirth, close monitoring is mandatory.

7 A. Viral hepatitis. Liver transplantation has been offered for an increasing array of indications over the last 10 years. Presently, the indications for transplantation are classified by the type of liver disease. Cirrhosis secondary to various forms of hepatitis, fulminant hepatitis B infection, and nonviral causes of hepatitis, such as autoimmune hepatitis, are the most common indications for liver transplantation. Transplantation for hepatitis B cirrhosis in patients with positive test results for HBsAg, HBeAg, or hepatitis B virus-DNA is associated with a high rate of recurrent disease in the absence of prophylactic treatment, as is transplantation for hepatitis C infection. These patients still have acceptable survival rates, however, and are currently considered appropriate candidates for transplantation. Recently, long term treatment with passive immunoprophylaxis and/or lamivudine has improved results in cases of active hepatitis B infection.

8 A 30-year-old male presents with a history of mild diarrhea with mucus and blood of 3 months duration. The stool cultures have been negative. On sigmoidoscopic investigation, the mucosa appears friable with signs of inflammation and bleeding. He has no fever but suffered a recent weight loss of 4.4 lb (2 kg). On examination, the abdomen is nontender and there is no hepatomegaly or splenomegaly. Laboratory investigations are shown.

Hemoglobin 12 g/dL (120 g/L)
WBC count 10,000/mm³ (10 × 10⁹/L)
Platelet count 410,000/mm³ (410 × 10⁹/L)
ESR 33 mm/hour
AST 120 U/L
ALT 180 U/L
ALP 1,540 U/L
Bilirubin 1.34 mg/dL (23 μmol/L)

i. What bowel disease must be considered?
ii. What further investigation must be undertaken?
iii. How shall the increases in AST, ALT, and ALP be interpreted?

9 This 7-year-old male has a history of jaundice since infancy. A heart murmur heard during the first year of life prompted a cardiac evaluation and echocardiography was consistent with a diagnosis of peripheral pulmonic stenosis. The patient is troubled by constant pruritus.

What does the appearance of the boy's face suggest (9)? What diagnosis is suspected?

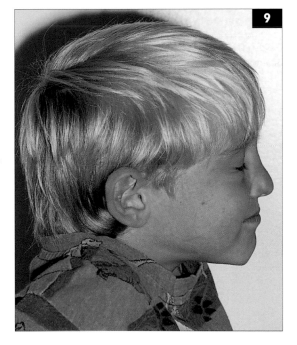

8 i. The absence of infection, the history of diarrhea with mucus and blood, and the appearance on sigmoidoscopy should suggest the possibility of inflammatory bowel disease, either ulcerative colitis or Crohn's disease.

ii. The patient should undergo a colonoscopic investigation with multiple biopsies in order to characterize the presumed inflammatory bowel disease and to determine the extent and distribution of the inflammation. This patient was confirmed as a case of ulcerative colitis with extensive bowel involvement.

iii. Some patients with severely active inflammatory bowel disease show pathological liver test results that subside when the bowel disease is in remission. On the other hand, 5% of patients with ulcerative colitis develop primary sclerosing cholangitis. The clinical priority in this case is to treat the patient's ulcerative colitis to induce a remission of the bowel disease. An ultrasound investigation of the liver should be undertaken in order to exclude any focal processes or dilation of the bile ducts. If the result of the ultrasound study is normal, liver tests should be repeated. If normalization occurs when the bowel disease is in remission, no further investigation will be necessary. The pathological liver test results can then be considered to be related to the activity of the colitis. The patient should, however, be screened regularly with liver tests every 3 months after normalization as primary sclerosing cholangitis may run a fluctuating course. If the liver tests remain abnormal an ERCP should be undertaken to clarify whether the patient has primary sclerosing cholangitis. This patient had a complete normalization of liver test results which remained normal for several years. No further investigations were required.

9 This patient has the typical face of Alagille's syndrome (also identified by different names including arteriohepatic dysplasia, syndromic paucity of interlobular bile ducts, and intrahepatic biliary hypoplasia). He has deep set eyes, frontal bossing, a bulbous tip of the nose, a down-turned mouth, a small mandible, and a pointed chin. Alagille's syndrome is a multisystem hereditary disorder that can first present with clinical symptoms involving the liver during infancy and early childhood. It has been recognized as a distinct syndrome for almost 30 years. It is seen throughout the world in many races and is more commonly reported in boys. It is the most common form of the familial intrahepatic cholestatic syndromes. The classic Alagille's syndrome involves five different findings which include: chronic cholestasis beginning in infancy with jaundice, itching, cholesterol deposits in the skin, and a liver biopsy which shows a paucity of interlobular bile ducts; congenital heart disease usually peripheral pulmonic stenosis although other heart disorders such as Tetrology of Fallot and coarctation of the aorta have been reported; bone defects usually 'butterfly' or hemi-vertebrae in the spine; eye findings of posterior embryotoxon which is an extra thickening of a line on the surface of the eye (Schwalbe's line) present from birth, or less common eye findings such as retinal pigment changes; and a typical face with deep set eyes, frontal bossing, a bulbous tip of the nose, a down-turned mouth, and a small mandible and pointed chin. Not all patients with Alagille's syndrome demonstrate all of the different findings. Recently, genetic analysis of the chromosomes of some patients with Alagille's syndrome has found a deletion in the short arm of chromosome 20.

10 A 62-year-old female cirrhotic patient consults because of abdominal pain, malaise, nausea, and vomiting. The patient denies fever or other symptomatology. Her cirrhosis had been diagnosed 8 years before after a first episode of ascites and she had been taking moderate doses of diuretics to control it. On examination moderate ascites is noted. Neither abdominal tenderness nor signs of hepatic encephalopathy are elicited. Laboratory investigations are shown.

Prothrombin time 21 seconds
Bilirubin 3 mg/dL (51.3 μmol/L)
Leukocytes 2.7 × 10³/mm³ (2.7 × 10⁹/L)
  (no leftward shift)
Ascitic fluid protein 1.5 g/dL (15 g/L)
Ascitic LDH 135 U/L
Ascitic amylase 200 U/L
Ascitic cell count 1,000 mm³ (1 × 10⁹/L)
  nucleated cells with 80%
  polymorphonuclear cells

i. What does the analysis of the ascitic fluid reveal?
ii. Should treatment be started?
iii. Should other investigations be undertaken?
iv. Could any prophylactic measures be recommended?

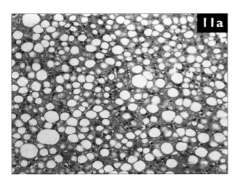
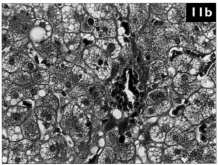

11 i. A 55-year-old white male with a long history of alcohol abuse is admitted for alcohol withdrawal. The patient began drinking 1 pint of vodka/day at age 25 years. Physical examination is within normal limits except for mild tender hepatomegaly. Laboratory investigations are shown.

i. What is the chance that this patient has liver fibrosis or cirrhosis?
ii. Comment on the liver biopsies shown (11a, b).
iii. What is the significance of the various liver test result abnormalities?
iv. What is the clinical significance of early fibrosis on liver biopsy?

Hemoglobin 14.2 g/dL (142 g/L)
Platelet count 240,000/mm³ (240 × 10⁹/L)
Prothrombin time 12.4 seconds
AST 88 U/L
ALT 28 U/L
Total protein 6.4 g/dL (64 g/L)
Albumin 3.8 g/dL (38 g/L)
ALP 120 U/L
GGTP 300 U/L
Total bilirubin 0.8 mg/dL (13.7 μmol/L)

10 i. This ascitic fluid is a transudate with low protein concentration as is usual in cirrhotic patients. However, the presence of ascitic fluid neutrophilia (polymorpho-nuclear count higher than $250/mm^3$ ($2.5 \times 10^8/L$)) points, with high sensitivity and specificity, to an infection. Taking into account the absence of an obvious intra-abdominal source of sepsis, the diagnosis would be spontaneous bacterial peritonitis.
ii. Even in the absence of clinical features of overt peritonitis or positive micro-biological cultures, empiric antibiotic treatment should be started immediately after neutrocytic ascitic fluid is noted. About 15% of the cases of spontaneous bacterial peritonitis are completely asymptomatic. Moreover, due to the low concentration of bacteria in the ascitic fluid, some cases of spontaneous bacterial peritonitis may have negative ascitic fluid cultures. Such cases are rare when more sensitive methods of ascitic fluid culture, such as blood culture bottles at the patient's bedside, are used. Cefotaxime is the preferred antibiotic for the initial empiric treatment of spontaneous bacterial peritonitis. No significant differences have been found between a short course (5 days) and long course (10 days) of treatment.
iii. It is important to check ascitic fluid polymorphonuclear counts after 48 hours of treatment in order to rule out treatment failure.
iv. Patients who survive an episode of spontaneous bacterial peritonitis are at high risk for developing recurrent episodes (almost 70% at 1 year) caused by aerobic Gram-negative enteric bacteria. Antibiotic prophylaxis, so-called selective intestinal decon-tamination, has shown to significantly reduce the probability of recurrence, and nor-floxacin 400 mg daily (at least during 1 year) is at present the most widely used strategy.

11 i. A dose response relationship exists between lifetime alcohol consumption and the risk of cirrhosis. The incidence of cirrhosis is significantly increased in men who consume over 40–60 g of ethanol daily. Among those who drink 180 g of alcohol daily for 8 years, approximately one third have biopsy confirmed cirrhosis or precirrhotic lesions. Fibrosis or cirrhosis may be present without physical or laboratory evidence.
ii. 11a depicts a liver biopsy demonstrating fatty liver with predominantly perivenular, macrovesicular steatosis. Trichrome staining in **11b** demonstrates fibrosis surrounding the terminal hepatic venule (perivenular fibrosis), individual hepatocytes (pericellular fibrosis), and sinusoids (perisinusoidal fibrosis).
iii. In early, precirrhotic alcoholic liver disease (fatty liver and perivenular fibrosis) routine liver tests are similar and are not helpful in predicting histological findings. Serum albumin and bilirubin levels as well as the prothrombin time are usually normal. GGTP levels are frequently elevated because of induction by alcohol. Aminotransferase levels are frequently mildly elevated (usually <250 U/L), and the ratio of AST to ALT is commonly >2.
iv. The presence of perivenular fibrosis predicts rapid progression to more severe stages of fibrosis (septal fibrosis to cirrhosis) within 2–4 years among those who continue to drink. By contrast, progression is infrequent and slow among patients with simple fatty liver whose alcohol consumption is comparable.

12 A 52-year-old female is referred for the evaluation of cryptogenic cirrhosis. She states that she usually drinks two glasses of wine during dinner and a 'night cap' or two before retiring at night. However, she adamantly denies drinking to excess or inebriation and displays no symptoms of dependence.

What is the possible role of alcohol in the development of this woman's liver disease?

13 A patient's variceal bleeding is controlled with endoscopic therapy (a band placed over the varix which preserves the polypoid nature of the varix until the ischemic tissue sloughs) and she has no further bleeding over the next 48 hours. Discussion with the patient's family reveals that she has had two recent admissions for alcohol detoxification. She has required 3 units of packed RBCs to stabilize her hematocrit at 32%.
i. What is the risk of this patient experiencing a recurrent variceal bleeding episode and what is the expected mortality for such an event?
ii. What is the greatest risk period for recurrent bleeding?

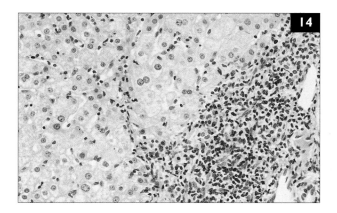

14 A 16-year-old Caucasian male born of a hepatitis B carrier mother was incidentally discovered to have serum HBsAg and elevated serum aminotransferase activities. He denied any symptoms. His liver was not palpable. Six months later he still had elevated ALT values. Laboratory investigations are shown. Abdominal ultrasound examination revealed a normal liver and spleen.
i. Describe the results of the liver biopsy (14).
ii. What is the utility of a liver biopsy in this condition?
iii. What is the diagnosis and natural history of this condition?

ALT 312 U/L
AST 164 U/L
Platelet count 250,000/mm³ (250 × 10⁹/L)
Bilirubin 1.1 mg/dL (18.8 μmol/L)
Albumin 4.3 g/dL (43 g/L)
Hepatitis B virus-DNA >1,000 pg/mL
Anti-HBc IgM absent
HBsAg present
HBeAg present
Anti-HCV absent

12 Women appear to be more susceptible than men to the toxic effects of alcohol. Whereas in men, a daily alcohol intake of 40–60 g results in a statistically significant increase in the incidence of cirrhosis, only 20 g (1–2 drinks) is required among women. In addition, progression to more severe liver fibrosis is more rapid among women, and the incidence of advanced chronic liver disease is higher among women than men with similar histories of alcohol abuse.

13 i. The risk of recurrent variceal hemorrhage, absent specific therapy, approaches 70% with a 30–50% mortality for each bleeding event. The risk is based on the patient's overall clinical status.
ii. The highest risk is within the first 6 months after control of the index bleed. The 50–70% rebleeding rate from esophageal varices is based on prospective studies of patients with variceal hemorrhage and data from medical control groups of randomized controlled trials to assess efficacy of pharmacologic, endoscopic, or surgical treatment for the prevention of recurrent variceal bleeding. Based on these data, all patients in whom the acute bleeding episode has been successfully controlled should have some form of medical or surgical therapy instituted as soon as possible to prevent recurrent bleeding. This should be instituted within 48 hours of control of the bleeding episode as the highest risk period for recurrent hemorrhage is the first 2 weeks after the index bleed.

14 i. The needle biopsy shows preservation of the lobular architecture. The portal area has a moderate degree of chronic inflammation with mononuclear cells. There is mild piecemeal necrosis, the parenchyma shows foci of necrosis, and several hepatocytes have uniformly pale eosinophilic cytoplasm (ground glass cytoplasm) indicating intracellular accumulation of HBsAg.
ii. In patients with persistently elevated aminotransferase activities, a liver biopsy helps to establish the diagnosis, to verify the etiology, to assess the severity of liver damage, to exclude other conditions, to guide the management, and to evaluate the effect of therapy.
iii. The diagnosis in this patient is chronic infection with hepatitis B virus causing moderate chronic active hepatitis. The presence of serum HBeAg, elevated ALT and AST, and high levels of hepatitis B virus -DNA in a carrier of HBsAg suggests infection with wild strains of hepatitis B virus. Genotypic varieties of hepatitis B virus with a point mutation in the precore region of hepatitis B virus do not secrete HBeAg. The time lag between exposure to and onset of clinical hepatitis is 6–26 weeks and the clinical expression of the infection is variable. Subclinical episodes of acute hepatitis are common as indicated by the large number of chronically infected patients who have no history of acute hepatitis. One to 3% of all acute cases progress to fulminant hepatic failure (50% mortality). The chance of developing chronic infection for the uncomplicated cases is over 50% during infancy and 3–8% in adulthood. Chronic inflammation may spontaneously subside leading to a healthy carrier state, or persist indefinitely causing mild to severe hepatic injury. In 20–30% of patients with chronic hepatitis, infection may progress to cirrhosis. The 5 year survival rate of patients with compensated cirrhosis is 72%.

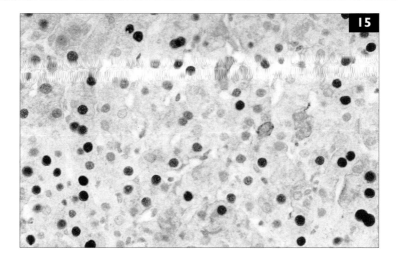

15 With regard to **14**, the patient's liver biopsy was stained for the presence of HBcAg using an immunoperoxidase method (**15**).
i. Comment on this biopsy result.
ii. What further investigations of the patient are recommended?
iii. What treatment is currently recommended for chronic hepatitis B infection?
iv. Can hepatitis B virus transmission be prevented?

16 A newborn patient is noted to have persistent indirect hyperbilirubinemia. The patient's urine is sampled and has a normal appearance.
    What management is suggested for this infant?

17 A 28-year-old, African–American male is referred for further evaluation of abnormal iron studies. He is known to have sickle cell anemia and has received multiple RBC transfusions for treatment of recurrent sickle cell crises and a poorly healing leg ulcer. From review of his old records, it appears that he has had at least 100 units of blood transfused over the past 8–10 years. The laboratory investigations are shown.
    How heavily iron-loaded is this individual?

Serum ferritin 5,780 ng/mL (103.46 μmol/L)
Transferrin saturation 85%
ALT 86 U/L
AST 75 U/L

15 i. The immunoperoxidase stain for HBcAg demonstrates numerous hepatocyte nuclei that are positive for the antigen (brown stain).

ii. Prospective monitoring of serum ALT and hepatitis B virus-DNA to identify factors predictive of a favorable response to interferon or lamivudine therapy, i.e. elevated ALT and low hepatitis B virus-DNA. Exclude autoimmunity and thyroid dysfunction which may contraindicate interferon therapy.

iii. Treatment to suppress virus replication. The ultimate goal is to eradicate hepatitis B virus and prolong patient survival. Interferon-alpha (or pegylated interferon, currently under investigation) administered for 4 months produces sustained disease remission in about 20% of patients. The most common beneficial response is the clearance of serum hepatitis B virus-DNA and HBeAg followed by seroconversion to anti-HBe and persistently normal ALT values. Lamivudine and adefovir have demonstrated efficacy in controlling virus replication and improving histology in patients with chronic hepatitis B.

iv. HBsAg carriers with HBeAg and elevated aminotransferase values are highly infectious. Vaccination of anti-HBs negative (susceptible) family members is necessary. Protected sex may prevent virus transmission in occasional partners.

16 No treatment is generally required for jaundice in full term infants. However, prolonged elevation of unconjugated bilirubin in full term newborns, or especially in premature infants, can result in neurologic injury and developmental delay. Exchange transfusion is indicated for infants with rapidly rising bilirubin levels or full term infants with serum unconjugated bilirubin levels >25–30 mg/dL (427–513 μmol/L), especially with hemolysis. Phototherapy is useful for infants with unconjugated hyperbilirubinemia resulting from nonhemolytic causes. If instituted early this may prevent rapid rises in bilirubin and the need for exchange transfusion. Phototherapy increases the energy of unconjugated bilirubin molecules allowing excretion of unconjugated bilirubin into the bile. Breast feeding jaundice has not been associated with development of kernicterus; thus many physicians recommend continued breast feeding. Curiously, discontinuation of breast feeding for a short period of 2–3 days causes a diminution of bilirubin levels which continues even if breast feeding is resumed. If Crigler–Najjar syndrome is being considered, administration of pheno-barbital is prudent to distinguish Crigler–Najjar types I and II. If hypothyroidism is identified in the etiology of unconjugated hyperbilirubinemia in a newborn, then thyroid replacement therapy is indicated.

17 He is likely to have at least 25 g of storage iron. (He has had 100 units of blood transfused with each unit containing about 250 mg of iron.) As a young man likely to need future blood transfusions, this patient represents a difficult problem. He is already significantly iron-loaded and no treatment for this has yet been given.

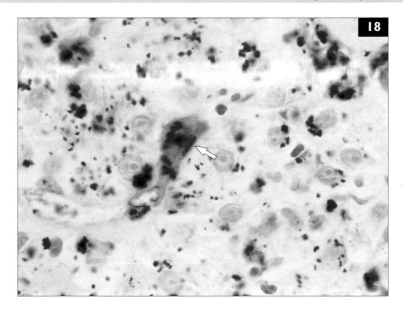

18 With regard to **17**, a liver biopsy was performed to determine the hepatic distribution of iron, the hepatic iron concentration, and the cause for the elevated aminotransferase values (**18**).
i. What is the distribution of iron in the liver biopsy?
ii. How should this patient be treated?

19 A 50-year-old male teacher has primary sclerosing cholangitis affecting both the intra- and extrahepatic biliary tracts which was diagnosed at 10 years of age. He also suffers from ulcerative colitis of 20 years duration. The colitis has been in remission for almost 10 years. During the last year, fatigue has slowly become more disabling. He has had jaundice for 1 year and pruritus causing sleeping problems. Laboratory investigations are shown.
   Which treatment options can be considered?

Hemoglobin 13 g/dL (130 g/L)
WBC count 7,000/mm³ (7 × 10⁹/L)
Platelet count 150,000/mm³ (150 × 10⁹/L)
ESR 15 mm/hour
AST 130 U/L
ALT 150 U/L
ALP 750 U/L
Bilirubin 9.1 mg/dL (156 µmol/L)
Albumin 2.8 g/dL (28 g/L)
Prothrombin time 12.5 seconds

18 i. The cellular distribution of iron in this patient shows iron predominantly in reticuloendothelial cells (Kupffer cells), with some in hepatocytes as well. The lobular distribution would be panlobular. Transfusional iron overload should be distinguished from hereditary hemochromatosis as there are differences in the mechanism whereby individuals become iron-loaded, the tissue and cellular sites of iron deposition, and the treatment. In individuals with hereditary hemochromatosis, the hepatic iron deposition is predominantly in hepatocytes with a periportal to central gradient. In transfusional iron overload, iron deposition is in reticulo-endothelial cells (Kupffer cells; 18, arrow) as well as in hepatocytes and is in a panlobular distribution rather than a periportal distribution.

ii. Treatment should be initiated with the iron-chelating drug deferoxamine. Whenever it appears that a patient with a dyserythropoietic anemia is going to require repeated blood transfusions, that patient should be considered for iron chelation therapy with deferoxamine in order to prevent or at least limit the degree of transfusional iron overload. Deferoxamine is administered either as a continuous subcutaneous infusion by way of a pump or by intravenous infusions given at night via a permanent indwelling catheter. When deferoxamine is administered, it is important to monitor for potential ophthalmologic or auditory complications.

19 There is currently no medical treatment with a proven positive effect on the survival of patients with primary sclerosing cholangitis, although there are studies indicating that ursodeoxycholic acid may affect liver biochemistry and histology favorably. It is, however, important to offer the patient symptomatic treatment. This patient has pruritus causing sleeping problems. It is always of importance when asking for pruritus to carefully analyze the impact of this symptom on the quality of life of the patient. Mild pruritus is common in patients with primary sclerosing cholangitis and usually requires no treatment. This patient could not sleep due to itching. Treatment with two doses per day of cholestyramine slowly resolved his symptoms. Primary sclerosing cholangitis is a disease with a highly variable course. Some patients may be asymptomatic for years whereas others may have a more aggressive form. Several attempts have been made to create a prognostic index. As yet, results have been variable. However, the presence of cirrhosis and a high bilirubin level, have been found to indicate a severe prognosis. In this patient a liver biopsy was carried out and biliary cirrhosis was detected. No focal process or dilation of the bile ducts was seen on ultrasound examination. Liver transplantation should be considered in every patient with advanced primary sclerosing cholangitis. With optimal timing of transplantation the 5 year survival rate for primary sclerosing cholangitis patients after the operation is 70–80%. This patient underwent liver transplantation without major complications. He is now doing well and returned to work as a full-time teacher.

20 A 72-year-old male presents with a 6 month history of increasing diarrhea and weight loss. His stools are pale and float. Three weeks before admission jaundice, pruritus, and dark urine developed. On examination multiple scratch marks, jaundice, and a mass in the right upper quadrant of the abdomen are noted.

i. What abnormality is shown on the ERCP (**20**)?
ii. What further investigations are indicated?
iii. What therapeutic options are available?

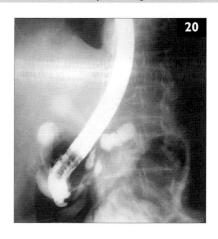

21 A 40-year-old female lawyer presents to the emergency room with a 2 day history of 'coffee ground' hematemesis and melena. She denies any past history of liver disease and states that she has 1–2 glasses of wine per night with dinner but rarely takes more. She does admit to some recent decrease in appetite and has lost 8–10 lb (3.6–4.5 kg) despite some recent increase in abdominal girth. On examination she is oriented but slightly confused, and has no asterixis. Her sclerae and skin are icteric. Her vital signs reveal orthostatic changes with her heart rate increasing from 90–120 beats/min and her blood pressure

Hematocrit 36%
Hemoglobin 10.3 g/dL (103 g/L)
WBC count 12,100/mm³ (12.1 × 10⁹/L)
Polymorphonuclear leukocytes 85%
Platelet count 90,000/mm³ (90 × 10⁹/L)
Prothrombin time 14.5 seconds
Bilirubin 4.6 mg/dL (78.7 μmol/L)
AST 150 U/L
ALT 90 U/L
ALP 230 U/L
Total protein 6.0 g/dL (60 g/L)
Albumin 2.4 g/dL (24 g/L)

dropping from 110/60–90/50 mmHg (14.7/8.0–12.0/6.7 kPa) in the sitting position. There are early signs of peripheral muscle wasting and she has 1–2 small spider angiomata over her upper back. Her lungs are clear to percussion and auscultation. She has a sinus tachycardia with a faint holosystolic murmur over the precordium. Abdominal examination reveals a protuberant abdomen with enlarged liver, palpable 10 cm (3.9 in) below the right costal margin and a spleen palpable 6 cm (2.5 in) below the left costal margin. She is estimated to have 2+ ascites and 1+ edema of her lower extremities. A rectal examination reveals black tarry stool. Laboratory investigations are shown. The viral serologies for hepatitis B virus and hepatitis C virus are negative. A blood ethanol level is 220 mg/dL (47.7 mmol/L). A drug screen is otherwise negative.

i. What are the most important initial measures to be taken by the emergency room physician for diagnosis and initial resuscitation of this patient?
ii. The gastroenterology consultant has been called. Should the emergency room physician initiate any specific treatment while awaiting endoscopy?

20 i. The ERCP shows obstruction in both the lower common bile duct and the head of the pancreas. This is a classical 'double-duct' sign of pancreatic carcinoma.

ii. Tests may be undertaken to confirm the diagnosis and to stage the disease with a view to defining operability. Histological confirmation can be obtained at the time of ERCP using brush cytology. The results are, however, often disappointing and in the best of hands a 50% positive yield can be expected. Alternatively percutaneous fine needle aspiration or true cut biopsy can be obtained under ultrasound or CT guidance. For patients in whom curative operations are being considered this may be unwise as it may seed tumor cells along the biopsy/aspiration tract. Staging of the tumor is initially based on ultrasound findings. Percutaneous ultrasound may show evidence of hepatic secondary deposits in which case further imaging is unnecessary. If the ultrasound scan does not show metastatic disease then a CT scan is a more sensitive modality. The findings of obvious metastatic disease or a tumor size >2–3 cm (>0.9–1.3 in) preclude further imaging as does encasement of enteric or portal vessels during the intravenous contrast phase of the examination. Patients may also be assessed by endoscopic ultrasound in which an ultrasound probe is combined with a modified endoscope. This visualizes the pancreas and may show evidence of tumor deposits within adjacent lymph nodes. There is little role for preoperative angiography as a staging modality but laparoscopy coupled with laparoscopic ultrasound is used before laparotomy in patients whose other screening tests suggest an operable tumor.

iii. Only 8–15% of adenocarcinomas of the pancreas are amenable to surgical resection and only the minority of these have long term survival. Therefore, the emphasis of treatment is upon relief of jaundice and pruritus by placement of stents within the biliary tree.

21 i. Initial management should include establishment of adequate venous access, replenishment of blood volume with packed RBCs and fresh frozen plasma and hydration to re-establish a euvolemic state. The patient should be evaluated for comorbid problems such as hepatic encephalopathy or sepsis.

ii. When the patient is suspected of having cirrhosis and portal hypertension, early initiation of pharmacologic therapy (vasopressin, somatostatin, octreotide, or terli-pressin) to control the bleeding decreases the morbidity and mortality associated with the bleeding episode. In an actively bleeding patient with ascites, initiation of prophylactic antibiotic therapy may be of value in preventing bacterial peritonitis.

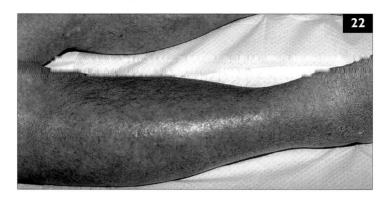

22 A 69-year-old female presents with fatigue, peripheral paraesthesis, arthralgias, leg edema, and purpura. On examination, the patient has moderate hypertension (170/110 mmHg (22.7/14.7 kPa)). Purpura involves both extremities and the left hemithorax. The liver and spleen are not palpable. Laboratory investigations are shown. Abdominal ultrasound shows ascitic fluid around the liver and in the pelvis. Chest X-rays show bilateral basal pleural effusions. A liver biopsy shows minimal inflammatory changes.

i. Comment on these physical findings in a patient with chronic hepatitis C (**22**).
ii. What is the diagnosis?
iii. Which further investigations should be performed?
iv. What is the pathogenesis and natural history of this condition?
v. Which treatment can be offered?

Hemoglobin 7.6 g/dL (76 g/L)
ALT normal
AST normal
Cryoglobulins present (410 mg/dL; IgG+A+M)
Total protein 5.1 g/dL (51 g/L)
Albumin 2.6 g/dL (26 g/L)
Creatinine 2.2 mg/dL (194.5 μmol/L)
BUN 67 mg/dL (urea 11.1 mmol/L)
HBsAg absent
Anti-HCV present
Urine showed micro/macro hematuria
Albuminuria 1.7 g/dL (17 g/L)
Rheumatoid factor positive

23 A 44-year-old male is being treated for chronic hypertension. His medical history is reported as 'unremarkable'. Laboratory investigations are shown.

What critical element of the history is lacking?

Hemoglobin 14.2 g/dL (142 g/L)
MCV 100.5 fL (mm³)
Platelet count 240,000/mm³ (240 × 10⁹/L)
Prothrombin time 12.4 seconds
AST 260 U/L
ALT 90 U/L
Total protein 6.4 g/dL (64 g/L)
Albumin 4.4 g/dL (44 g/L)
ALP 120 U/L
GGTP 300 U/L
Total bilirubin 0.8 g/dL (13.7 μmol/L)

22 i. This picture shows extensive purpura on the extremities as a result of vasculitis. In chronic liver diseases purpura may also result from thrombocytopenia.

ii. Hepatitis C related mixed cryoglobulinemia (type 3) leading to nephrotic syndrome.

iii. Quantative assessment of serum hepatitis C virus-RNA, nonorgan-specific serum antibodies, thyroid antibodies and function, and serum ferritin, iron, and transferrin. These investigations are aimed at assessing the presence of autoimmune reactions and levels of hepatitis C virus replication. Autoimmune reactions may contraindicate treatment with interferon.

iv. Approximately 50% of chronic carriers of hepatitis C virus produce detectable amounts of cryoglobulins. However, only a minority of patients develop clinical and, or, laboratory signs of vasculitis including purpura or glomerulonephritis. Cryoglobulins are serum proteins comprised of immunoglobulins that precipitate in the cold. Three different patterns of cryoglobulinemia are recognized. Types 2 and 3 are mixed forms. The former is a mixture of polyclonal immunoglobulin of different classes and an IgM monoclonal component that has rheumatoid factor activity. Type 3 cryoglobulins are exclusively polyclonal with an IgM component with rheumatoid factor activity. Mixed cryoglobulins accompany a diverse group of infectious and noninfectious conditions. Initial reports suggested a significant association between type 2 and 3 cryoglobulinemia and hepatitis B virus. In several countries, most cases of mixed cryoglobulinemia appear to be related to hepatitis C viral infection, and occur more commonly in females. The disappearance of cryoglobulinemia with successful interferon therapy was taken as support of the pathogenic role of hepatitis C virus in this syndrome. This condition is characterized by arthralgias, vasculitis, purpura, neuropathy, and glomerulonephritis.

v. Hypertension was successfully controlled with daily administration of antihypertensives. Treatment with interferon-alpha at doses of 3 MU three times weekly for 12 months led to disappearance of serum hepatitis C viral-RNA, an increase in total protein and hemogloblin (7.5 g/dL [75 g/L] and 11 g/dL [110 g/L], respectively), reduction of creatinine to 1.7 mg/dL (150 µmol/L), cryocrit to 0.3%, and proteinuria to 0.2 g/dL (2 g/L). Weakness, arthralgias, paraesthesias, purpura, and edema disappeared following therapy. Although the use of ribavirin is problematic in patients with renal insufficiency, the use of pegylated interferons will likely replace standard interferons.

23 In many developed countries alcohol consumption poses significant long term risks for a relatively large proportion of the population. In the United Kingdom, 25% of men consume more than 210 g of alcohol per week and 8% of women more than 150 g (each drink is approximately 12–14 g of alcohol). As little as 1–2 drinks/day significantly increases the risk of cirrhosis. Because early detection of significant medical conditions is critical, recognition of problem drinking is important. However, patients are infrequently asked about alcohol consumption during the medical examination, and, as a result the problem, is commonly not identified. Excessive alcohol consumption complicates many medical conditions. In this case, it would impair blood pressure control.

24 A 27-year-old water engineer returns from working in West Africa and 3 weeks later develops low grade fever, malaise, and jaundice. Laboratory investigations are shown.
i. What is the differential diagnosis?
ii. How may the diagnosis be made?

Hemoglobin 13.4 g/dL (134 g/L)
WBC count 4,000/mm³ (4.0 × 10⁹/L)
  with lymphocytosis on a differential count.
AST 1,010 U/L
ALT 1,538 U/L
Bilirubin 4.68 mg/dL (80 µmol/L)
Albumin 4.2 g/dL (42 g/L)
ALP 280 U/L
Prothrombin time 13 seconds

Hemoglobin 12.7 g/dL (127 g/L)
Platelet count 82,000/mm³
  (82 × 10⁹/L)
Prothrombin time 14 seconds
ALT 50 U/L
AST 60 U/L
Ceruloplasmin 40 mg/dL
  (400 mg/L)

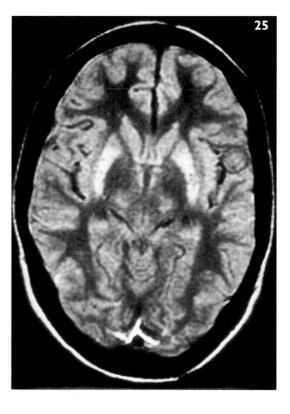

25 A 21-year-old female presents with dysarthria, dysphagia, slurring of her speech, and tremors which had progressively worsened over the course of a year. Physical examination is remarkable for the above neurologic findings, gait abnormality, and splenomegaly. An MRI scan of the brain was undertaken (**25**). Laboratory investigations are shown.
i. What does the combination of neurologic symptoms and findings, the MRI scan of the brain, and presence of liver disease suggest?
ii. What studies are needed to confirm the diagnosis?

24 i. The differential diagnosis is wide, but it is most likely to be infective. Viral infection including hepatitis A, B, C, D, and E may all cause an acute icteric illness (D only in the presence of chronic B infection). Epstein–Barr virus, CMV, varicella, herpes simplex types 1 and 2, paramyxovirus, coxsackievirus, rubella, flavivirus (causing yellow fever), Marburg virus, and the zoonotic arenavirus (causing lassa fever) can also result in this clinical picture. Rickettsial infection by *Coxiella burnetti* causes Q fever. Possible bacterial causes include leptospirosis, with tuberculosis, brucellosis, and syphilis as rarer cases. Protozoal infection can result in toxoplasmosis. Alcohol is unlikely to be the sole cause, as the enzyme rise of ALT and AST is too high for alcoholic hepatitis alone. Drugs, for example, paracetamol and salicylates, antibiotics (tetracycline, rarely penicillin, and sulphonamides), and nonsteroidal anti-inflammatory agents are the most likely to be implicated in this context.

ii. Although many of the infective agents above produce the same picture, the incubation period, prodrome of malaise, jaundice, and a history of water contact suggest hepatitis A. The diagnosis is made on serology. Hepatitis A may be diagnosed from the presence of specific IgM anti-HAV antibodies, or total specific anti-HAV antibodies (including both IgM and IgG). Most patients are IgM positive by the onset of their symptoms, and remain positive for 3–6 months. IgG antibodies to hepatitis A virus persist for years, and immunity following infection is lifelong. Diagnosis of the other infective agents listed above is also serological.

25 i. The combination of neurologic symptoms and liver disease should prompt a search for the unifying diagnosis of Wilson's disease. Wilson's disease is an autosomal recessive disorder in which copper accumulates first in the liver, then later in extrahepatic sites. Untreated, the disease leads to progressive symptoms and liver failure. The MRI scan of the brain, remarkable for hyperintensity in the region of the basal ganglia, is caused by the increased metal content of the tissue. This finding alone is suggestive of Wilson's disease.

ii. The possibility of Wilson's disease should be excluded by a combination of clinical and laboratory studies. The patient should undergo a slit-lamp examination to exclude the presence of Kayser–Fleischer rings, corneal deposits of copper in Descemet's membrane. In Wilson's disease, Kayser–Fleischer rings are almost invariably present at the time neurologic symptoms are manifest, as is cirrhosis of the liver. A serum ceruloplasmin oxidase activity should be obtained as serum levels of the activity of this protein are reduced in 90% of patients with Wilson's disease. It may also be reduced in 20% of asymptomatic carriers (heterozygotes). The combination of Kayser–Fleischer rings and a reduced serum ceruloplasmin activity is adequate to establish a diagnosis of Wilson's disease. With patients symptomatic for neurologic Wilson's disease, studies of the brain, either MRI or CT scans, reveal abnormalities which are not confined to the basal ganglia. Proton density MRI may better indicate the presence of metal deposition. The abnormalities noted on brain scans may not correlate with the degree of clinical symptoms and are not predictive of the degree of recovery when specific treatment is initiated.

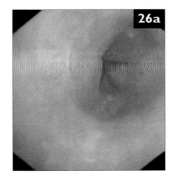

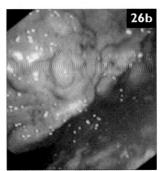

26 A 14-year-old male has portal hypertension from congenital hepatic fibrosis. He has suffered two variceal bleeds. His esophagus and stomach at endoscopy are shown (**26a, b**). He has no encephalopathy and is in good nutritional condition. Examination reveals spider angiomata and a caput medusa, but no asterixis. Laboratory investigations are shown. He is best managed with which of the following:

Prothrombin time 12 seconds
Bilirubin 1.5 mg/dL (25.65 μmol/L)
Albumin 4.5 g/dL (45 g/L)

A Distal splenorenal shunt.
B Esophageal variceal banding.
C Endoscopic sclerotherapy.
D Liver transplantation.

27 A 45-year-old Caucasian male presented with upper abdominal discomfort. Physical examination was unremarkable. Blood tests were notable for mildly elevated aminotransferase values (ALT 85 U/L and AST 55 U/L). A CT scan of the abdomen was performed (**27**).
i. What does the CT scan show?
ii. What is the differential diagnosis?
iii. Are there risk factors for hepatocellular carcinoma which can be evaluated clinically in this patient?

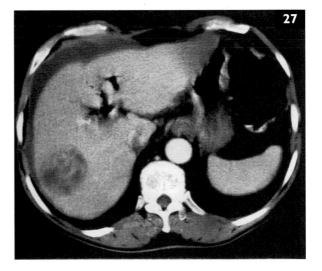

26 A. Distal splenorenal shunt. Congenital hepatic fibrosis is usually a sporadic disease, but it can also occur as a familial form with autosomal recessive inheritance. It is a disorder of development of the bile ducts in which normal hepatic lobules are surrounded with fibrous bands often containing partially developed bile ductules. It is associated with portal hypertension but does not usually progress to cirrhosis. This patient has portal hypertension but evidence of normal hepatic synthetic function. The clinical examination and laboratory test results reveal this patient to be Child's classification A; with good nutrition, no ascites, no encephalopathy, normal bilirubin, and normal albumin levels. Treatment must be directed at the portal hypertension alone, and therefore liver transplantation is unnecessary. Endoscopic sclerotherapy and variceal banding have been shown to be effective in the setting of esophageal varices but are not effective in the long term control of hemorrhage from gastric varices. Shunting procedures are both effective and safe for control of variceal hemorrhage when performed in patients with Child's class A synthetic function. Both portocaval shunt and distal splenorenal shunt are options for this patient, but the splenorenal shunt is most effective with the lowest morbidity for control of gastric varices. A portocaval shunt is the preferred operation for very small children. The patient is best managed with the distal splenorenal shunt. Placement of a TIPS achieves lowered portal pressures but has a high rate of shunt thrombosis (50% at 1 year) and is not a suitable option in a patient with a long life expectancy.

27 i. The CT scan shows a 5 cm (2 in) solid mass in the right lobe of the liver. The liver is normal sized with smooth borders. There is no intra-abdominal adenopathy and the hepatic vessels appear patent. There is no ascites or splenomegaly.
ii. The differential diagnosis of a solitary hepatic mass includes primary malignant neoplasms of the liver such as hepatocellular carcinoma, cholangiocarcinoma, biliary tract adenocarcinoma, angiosarcoma, and epithelioid hemangioendothelioma. Metastatic tumors of the liver are usually multifocal, but metastatic melanoma and colorectal adenocarcinoma can present as solitary lesions. Also included in the differential diagnosis are benign tumors such as hepatocellular adenoma, focal nodular hyperplasia, nodular regenerative hyperplasia, hemangioma, and cystadenoma.
iii. Hepatocellular carcinoma usually develops in patients with chronic liver disease of any etiology. Clinical evidence for chronic liver disease can be detected on physical examination (spider angiomata, ascites, hepatomegaly, splenomegaly, gynecomastia, and testicular atrophy), on blood tests (elevated biochemical liver tests, decreased albumin, thrombocytopenia, and elevated prothrombin time), and nodular heterogeneous liver on CT scan. Specific etiologies can be detected by viral hepatitis serologies (HBsAg, hepatitis C antibody), autoimmune markers (antimitochondrial, antismooth muscle, and antinuclear antibodies), serum ferritin and transferrin saturation, and alpha-1-antitrypsin phenotype. Hepatocellular carcinoma may sometimes develop in the absence of chronic liver disease but in association with the use of anabolic steroids, oral contraceptives, and exposure to thorotrast, a radiographic contrast agent used in the 1950s.

28 With regard to the patient in 27:

i. Is an elevated serum alphafetoprotein level pathognomonic for hepatocellular carcinoma?

The patient was found to have a normal serum alphafetoprotein level.

ii. What test would you order to produce a definitive diagnosis?

iii. Describe the pathology of hepatocellular carcinoma (28a–d).

iv. A definitive diagnosis of hepatocellular carcinoma was made. How would you treat this patient?

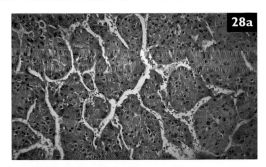

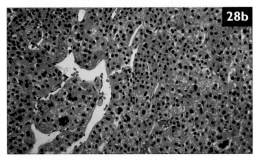

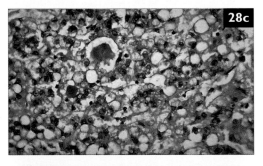

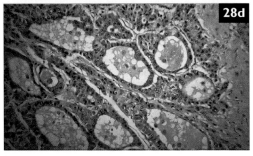

28 i. Alphafetoprotein, a product of fetal and regenerating liver, is detectable in the serum at low levels (<10 ng/mL) in normal adults and children over the age of 1 year. Up to 80% of patients with hepatocellular carcinoma have elevated serum levels. The positive predictive value of a serum level >400 ng/mL is more than 95%. A rising serum alphafetoprotein of any value should, however, trigger a search for hepatocellular carcinoma, particularly in patients with chronic liver disease. Note again that 20% of patients with hepatocellular carcinoma do not have an elevated serum alphafetoprotein. Other conditions where elevated serum alphafetoprotein levels are seen include acute hepatitis (<400 ng/mL), nonseminomatous testicular carcinoma with embryonal elements (associated with elevated serum levels of beta-human chorionic gonadotropin), and gastric adenocarcinoma.

ii. Radiologic imaging may be helpful. Ultrasound and CT scans are both sensitive in detecting small lesions and assessing cirrhosis. When combined with duplex Doppler, ultrasound can detect malignant vascular thromboses and reversal of portal vein flow. Nuclear scintigraphy, particularly when coupled with single proton emission CT imaging, is helpful in the diagnosis of hemangiomas. MRI scans generally do not provide additional information after ultrasound and CT scan, but may help to distinguish benign lesions such as regenerative nodules and hemangiomas from hepatocellular carcinoma. The gold standard for definitive diagnosis of hepatocellular carcinoma is histological evaluation of a core biopsy of the mass. A core biopsy can be obtained under ultrasound or CT guidance. Alternatively, percutaneous aspiration of the tumor for cytological examination can be performed with a fine needle. However, hepatocellular carcinoma, particularly the well differentiated histological type, may appear benign on cytological evaluation, as a disruption of the tissue architecture may be the only sign of malignancy on histological evaluation. Immuno-histochemical stains for alphafetoprotein, carcinoembryonic antigen (a canalicular pattern is seen in hepatocellular carcinoma), and cytokeratin (negative in hepato-cellular carcinoma) may be helpful in difficult cases.

iii. The pathology of hepatocellular carcinoma ranges from well differentiated (**28a**) to poorly differentiated (**28b**), from clear cell (**28c**) to spindle cell variants. Hepato-cellular carcinoma may also assume a 'pseudoglandular' pattern (**28d**), which should be distinguished from the glandular features of adenocarcinomas.

iv. Hepatocellular carcinoma can be treated by surgical resection as long as the integrity of vascular and biliary structures can be maintained. Its regenerative capacity allows up to 80% of a normal liver to be resected. A chronically diseased liver may have inadequate function to allow resection, and may not be able to regenerate sufficiently. Patients with chronic liver disease and hepatocellular carcinoma should, therefore, be assessed for adequate residual hepatic function before resection. Several parameters indicate hepatic reserve, including the degree of liver dysfunction based both on markers of synthetic function (albumin and prothrombin time) and on biochemical liver tests, especially bilirubin; and also on the proportion of liver to be resected.

29 A 35-year-old male presents with a history of primary sclerosing cholangitis and ulcerative colitis of 5 years duration. The colitis was characterized by episodes of bleeding and diarrhea. There is evidence of involvement of both the intra- and extrahepatic biliary passages. A liver biopsy undertaken 1 year previously showed early changes with inflammation and fibrosis in the periportal regions. Over the years the patient has mostly been asymptomatic, although there have been

Hemoglobin 13 g/dL (130 g/L)
WBC count 9,000/mm³ (9 × 10⁹/L)
Platelet count 350,000/mm³ (350 × 10⁹/L)
ESR 15 mm/hour
AST 92 U/L
ALT 104 U/L
ALP 430 U/L
Bilirubin 3.68 mg/dL (63 µmol/L)
Albumin 3 g/dL (30 g/L)
Prothrombin time 17 seconds

episodes of upper right abdominal pain and itching. Lately, he has experienced repeated episodes of abdominal pain; he has also noted jaundice. The colitis has been kept in remission for several years with olsalazine treatment. However, lately the patient has had 2–3 pale loose stools every day, without rectal bleeding. He has lost 8.8 lb (4 kg) in weight over the preceding 6 months. Laboratory investigations are shown.
i. Why is the patient passing pale stools and losing weight?
ii. What further investigations should be considered?

30 A 54-year-old, white male is seen for evaluation of arthralgias. He has taken over-the-counter nonsteroidal anti-inflammatory agents in the past with intermittent relief of symptoms. He complains of pain in the joints of both hands, in his knees, and occasionally in his hips. A screening blood chemistry panel is normal except that his transferrin saturation is increased at 92%. His CBC is normal. Radiographs of the affected joints show normal hip X-rays and chondrocalcinosis in the knees. Films of the hands are shown (30a, b).

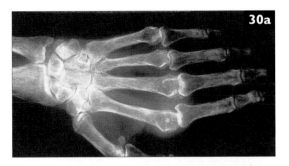

30a

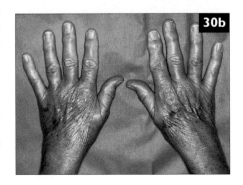

30b

i. What are the typical joints affected in hemochromatosis?
ii. How commonly do patients with hemochromatosis present with joint symptoms?
iii. How responsive are the joint symptoms to phlebotomy therapy?

29 i. If the patient has decolored fatty stools and, or, significant biliary outflow problems indicating malabsorption of fat, pancreatic problems must be suspected. Celiac disease should not be forgotten, as there is increased prevalence in primary sclerosing cholangitis. This may well explain the decreased prothrombin level and the low serum albumin.

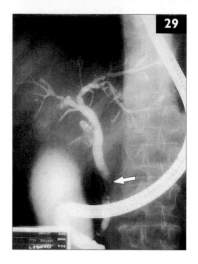

ii. An ultrasound investigation should be undertaken to reveal possible dilation of the bile ducts and an ERCP to find out whether significant extrahepatic biliary strictures are present (**29**, arrow). This patient has a dominant bile duct structure. As 10–20% of all patients with primary sclerosing cholangitis develop cholangiocarcinoma, brush cytology was taken to exclude malignancy. Duodenal biopsy should be carried out to exclude celiac disease. A balloon dilation was undertaken and the lumen became widened to 2 mm (0.08 in) afterwards, allowing free passage of contrast. After the dilation the jaundice disappeared and the bowel function returned to normal. Pancreatography revealed no abnormality, although 10–30% of primary sclerosing cholangitis patients have coexisting pancreatic strictures. Pancreatic exocrine insufficiency is rare, but should be considered. Dilation of the biliary tree in primary sclerosing cholangitis should be undertaken if the patient has a history of significant obstruction with jaundice, malabsorption, or pain. If the patient has cirrhosis or signs of liver decompensation a liver transplantation should be considered. Treatment of fat soluble vitamin deficiency should be carried out. Bone densitometry may indicate the need for specific treatment with agents such as bisphosphonates to reduce bone loss.

30 i. The second and third metacarpophalangeal joints of the hands are the most commonly affected in hereditary hemochromatosis. However, the joints of the wrists, shoulders, hips, and knees can be affected. The most common radiographic findings are chondrocalcinosis, joint space narrowing, subchondral cyst formation, and osteopenia.

ii. Joint symptoms are one of the most common presenting symptoms for patients with hereditary hemochromatosis. In one series published in 1980, arthralgias accounted for the most common presenting symptom in patients with hemochromatosis, accounting for 54% of patients. With more patients being identified by routine chemistry screening panels, the prevalence of joint symptoms is decreasing.

iii. Unfortunately, the arthropathy of hemochromatosis usually does not respond to phlebotomy therapy. Even after patients have become iron depleted, they still may have symptoms of joint pain. Patients may require continued use of nonsteroidal anti-inflammatory agents and occasionally intra-articular injections of corticosteroids are necessary.

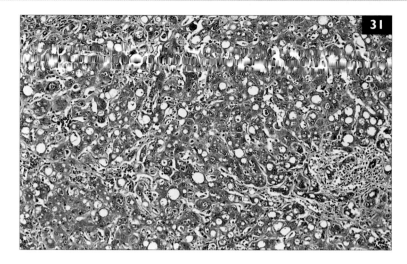

31 i. Why should a liver biopsy be performed in the evaluation of a patient suspected of having Wilson's disease?

ii. What treatment should be given to the patient whose liver biopsy is shown above (31)?

32 A group of medical students submitted to a serologic profile to screen for hepatitis B virus infection. The following patterns were identified:

	HBsAg	anti-HBs	IgG anti-HBc	IgM anti-HBc	HBeAg	anti-HBe	Hepatitis B virus DNA
A	–	+	+	–	–	+	–
B	+	–	+	–	–	+	–
C	–	+	–	–	–	–	–
D	+	–	–	+	+	–	+
E	+	–	+	–	–	+	+

Match the serologic pattern with the diagnoses listed below and explain why the answer is correct.

i. Acute hepatitis B.

ii. Chronic hepatitis B (wild type).

iii Chronic hepatitis B (precore mutant).

iv. Previous infection with immunity.

v. Previous hepatitis B vaccination.

31 i. If doubt remains as to the diagnosis of Wilson's disease, a liver biopsy should be obtained for histologic examination and quantitative copper determination. The liver biopsy shown (**31**) has been stained with H&E and demonstrates granular deposition of copper (brown). Steatosis is present, as is common. Fibrosis is seen in portal areas. Hepatic copper concentrations of more than 250 µg/g dry weight of liver are consistent with Wilson's disease, but may rarely be found in association with cholestatic disorders or idiopathic copper toxicosis syndromes. Clinical history and histologic evaluation readily distinguish between these disorders. If liver biopsy is difficult to obtain or contraindicated, then a 24 hour urine for copper quantitation can also help confirm the diagnosis. Copper levels exceeding 100 µg/24 hours are seen frequently in symptomatic patients.

ii. Treatment specific for Wilson's disease should be initiated. Penicillamine, a copper chelating agent would be the treatment of choice for symptomatic patients. With appropriate monitoring, the presence of a reduced platelet count does not preclude the use of this drug. On initiation of therapy the patient should be monitored for fever or rash, thrombocytopenia, proteinuria, and a lupus-like syndrome. The neurologic and hepatic abnormalities caused by Wilson's disease may take months to resolve. If treatment is delayed, the neurologic disease may be irreversible.

Once the diagnosis of Wilson's disease is established, screening of other family members must be performed.

32 i. Pattern D is characteristic of acute hepatitis B based on the presence of HBsAg and IgM anti-HBc. In addition, patients with acute hepatitis B will have active viral replication with detectable HBeAg and hepatitis B virus-DNA.

ii. Pattern B is characteristic of chronic hepatitis B infection with the usual, wild type of hepatitis B virus. The presence of HBsAg and IgG anti-HBc is compatible with chronic, rather than acute, hepatitis B virus infection. The anti-HBs does not reflect immunity when present with HBsAg; it is found in up to 20% of patients with chronic hepatitis B and is a heterotypic antibody. The absence of HBeAg and hepatitis B virus-DNA indicates a nonreplicative stage of chronic hepatitis B.

iii. Pattern E is characteristic of chronic hepatitis B infection with the precore mutant type of hepatitis B virus. The presence of a HBsAg and IgG anti-HBc is compatible with chronic hepatitis. B. The finding of detectable hepatitis B virus DNA but not HBeAg is the characteristic serologic finding that indicates the presence of a precore mutant hepatitis B virus. In addition, anti-HBe is detectable, and patients characteristically have moderately elevated aminotransferase activities.

iv. Pattern A shows the presence of anti-HBs and IgG anti-HBc, which indicates natural immunity. In addition, anti-HBe is also usually present. Some patients will lose detectable anti-HBs and anti-HBe and will only have IgG anti-HBc as evidence of prior hepatitis B virus infection.

v. Pattern C is characteristic of hepatitis B virus vaccination, which results in the development of only anti-HBs and not IgG anti-HBc which is seen in natural immunity.

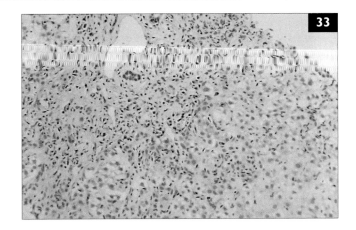

33 A 57-year-old female was investigated for marked fatigue. Laboratory investigations are shown.

She had been taking metoprolol for several years for essential hypertension. Routine blood tests had revealed normal aminotransferase activity. Because of symptomatic osteoarthritis, diclofenac had been added 3 months earlier. She was referred to a gastro-enterologist. Physical examination was unremark-able except for areas of cutaneous depigmentation. No findings suggestive of chronic liver disease were found. A percutaneous liver biopsy was performed (33).

Hematocrit 40%
AST 220 U/L
ALT 335 U/L
ANA 1:320
Antithyroglobulin antibodies 1:160
Bilirubin 1.0 mg/dL (17.1 μmol/L)
ALP 100 U/L

i. What does the biopsy reveal? What is the likely diagnosis?
ii. What is the significance of the physical and laboratory findings to the diagnosis?
iii. What is the pathogenesis of this condition?
iv. What is the prognosis of this condition?

34 An 18-year-old female presents to her general practitioner with a 2 week history of increasing jaundice and lethargy. She is not on medication. A diagnosis of 'acute hepatitis' is made but over a 10 week period there has been no improvement and the jaundice and symptoms of lethargy persist. On examination, the liver is enlarged 4 cm (1.6 in) below the right coastal margin but there are no other positive physical findings. Her medical history reveals she has had two similar episodes over the last 2 years both of which subsided spontaneously within a few weeks. Laboratory investigations are shown.

AST 660 U/L
Bilirubin 7.07 mg/dL (121 μmol/L)
ALP 100 U/L

What additional laboratory investigations should be undertaken on referral?

33 i. The liver histology shows chronic active hepatitis with autoimmune-like features including prominent disruption of the limiting plate (present diffusely in all periportal zones) and significant numbers of plasma cells. This patient had been receiving diclofenac for 3 months when she presented with serologic (positive for antinuclear antibodies) and histologic features of autoimmune chronic active hepatitis. The likely diagnosis is diclofenac-induced hepatitis with features of autoimmune hepatitis.

ii. The patient had other evidence of an autoimmune disorder, vitiligo (areas of cutaneous depigmentation) and high-titer antithyroglobulin antibodies.

iii. The molecular basis by which diclofenac leads to liver injury is unknown. It appears to involve the modification of tissue proteins by reactive metabolites of diclofenac. Some studies suggest a hypersensitivity basis for the toxicity, while others favour a metabolic mechanism. Either mechanism of cell damage could be attributed to the covalent modification of tissue proteins by reactive metabolites of dilocfenac. The metabolic mechanism of toxicity might be caused by the alteration of a vital cellular function as a consequence of protein adduct formation. The hypersensitivity mechanism of toxicity might be caused by an immune response against covalent adducts (neoantigens) that are displayed on the cell surface of hepatocytes.

iv. The injury usually subsides within 4 weeks after the drug has been stopped. A number of drugs have been incriminated in the production of chronic necroinflammatory hepatic disease that may resemble either viral (e.g. isoniazid) or autoimmune chronic hepatitis (e.g. dantrolene, methyldopa, nitrofurantoin, oxyphenisatin, and propylthiouracil). The autoimmune chronic hepatitis-like reaction resembles so called lupoid hepatitis in its histologic and clinical features. There is a striking female preponderance among patients. The histologic lesion is characterized by dramatic portal and periportal inflammation composed of lymphocytes, plasma cells, and often eosinophils. A cardinal histologic characteristic is the extension of the inflammation, commonly accompanied by fibrous strands, into the periportal parenchyma, surrounding individual degenerating cells and groups of cells (interface hepatitis). Diclofenac, a widely used nonsteroidal anti-inflammatory drug, is a derivative of phenylacetic acid. Most cases occur within 3 months of initiating therapy and typically present with anorexia, nausea, vomiting, abdominal pain, tender hepatomegaly, and jaundice. Complete clinical recovery usually occurs with the discontinuance of diclofenac, but 10% of the reported cases have been fatal.

34 The illness is clearly 'hepatic' and this influences the investigative approach. A CBC and prothrombin time should be undertaken. These help to determine if a liver biopsy is contraindicated. The prothrombin time is a valuable test of 'liver function'. Viral hepatitis screening including anti-HAV, HBsAg, and antibody to hepatitis C should be obtained. Epstein–Barr virus serology should be determined as all these viral infections may give a similar clinical picture. Ceruloplasmin levels should be tested to exclude Wilson's disease. Alpha-1-antitrypsin deficiency produces the histological features of chronic active hepatitis and needs to be ruled out. Autoantibodies and immunoglobulin tests should include smooth muscle and antinuclear antibodies.

35 The patient in 34 has a positive smooth muscle antibody test 1:100, the antinuclear antibodies >1:400, and the gamma globulin is 6.6 g/dL (66 g/L), mainly IgG (1.6 g/dl [16 g/L]). All virological tests are negative. A diagnosis of autoimmune hepatitis is considered and a liver biopsy is advised. However, fearing horrid stories of possible complications she is very reluctant to undergo this procedure. Her local physician cannot make a good case for it either.

Why is a biopsy important?

36 A 13-year-old female presents with jaundice and a painful right upper quadrant mass. The serum liver tests show a cholestatic pattern. Transabdominal ultrasound shows a grossly dilated common bile duct.
i. What does the ERCP show (36)?
ii. Is the pancreatic duct normal?
iii. What is the prognosis?
iv. What treatment is required?

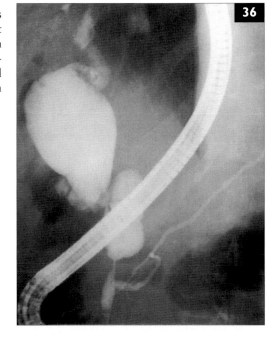

37 Simple screening instruments have been developed to detect problem drinking, including the CAGE questionnaire (right).

When problem drinking is detected, what interventions are available to reduce alcohol consumption?

The CAGE questionnaire for alcoholism:

C Have you ever felt you ought to **C**ut down on drinking?
A Have people **A**nnoyed you by criticizing your drinking?
G Have you ever felt bad or **G**uilty about your drinking?
E Have you ever had a drink first thing in the morning to steady your nerves or get rid of a hangover (**E**ye opener)?

35 The biopsy is necessary to confirm the histological picture of chronic active hepatitis. It also acts as a baseline for subsequent biopsies. The biopsy helps predict a more accurate prognosis. The survival rate is lower if the patient already has cirrhosis. The risks associated with subsequent pregnancy are considerably greater if there is established cirrhosis. If fibrosis or cirrhosis are present then chronicity is confirmed. The tissue sample can also be used for assessment of copper to exclude Wilson's disease. (See also **48**.)

36 i. Cystic dilation of the common bile duct is consistent with choledochal cyst. The majority of choledochal cysts involve the common bile duct; occasionally the cystic duct or the intraduodenal part of the bile duct may be involved. Most cases arise in females and the classical presentation is that of abdominal pain, obstructive jaundice, and an abdominal mass. Cholangitis can occur because of associated common bile duct debris. Abdominal pain may occur as a consequence of tortion of the cyst. Cysts occasionally lead to liver abscess formation. They can sometimes rupture, cause pancreatitis, or obstruct the portal vein.
ii. While the pancreatic duct is not obstructed in this case there is anomalous drainage to the lower part of the common bile duct. This is a common accompaniment of the anomaly that may cause acute pancreatitis.
iii. Choledochal cysts are strongly associated with cholangiocarcinoma. Approximately 14% of patients with untreated cysts over the age of 20 develop these tumors. In addition choledochal cysts left untreated may lead to secondary biliary cirrhosis consequent upon biliary obstruction and recurrent episodes of sepsis.
iv. Diagnosis of choledochal cysts is followed by strong consideration of resection as incomplete excision risks malignant transformation. In cases where a surgical resection is impossible hepaticojejunostomy and partial excision is an alternative.

37 When excessive alcohol consumption is detected, simple advice that includes information about how to abstain or reduce consumption and the suggestion to keep a drinking diary is often effective. Two drugs are also available to maintain sobriety: disulfiram and naltrexone. Disulfiram produces a highly aversive episode of flushing, weakness, and nausea and, occasionally, hypotension in patients who drink alcohol. The episode is caused by increasing circulating acetaldehyde levels via the inhibition of aldehyde dehydrogenase activity and the lack of an appropriate norepinephrine response because of inhibition of dopamine beta oxidation. Only supervised ingestion of the drug (250–500 mg/day) leads to prolonged (6 month) abstinence in approximately half of patients. As the drug possesses significant toxicity, its use should be restricted to patients who are motivated to stay sober, who understand the risk of drinking while using the drug, and who are not pregnant. It should not be given to patients in whom hypotensive episodes are hazardous, such as those with significant cardiovascular disease. Naltrexone, an oral opiate antagonist, is a recent alternative to disulfiram. Naltrexone (50 mg daily) when combined with psychotherapy decreases craving for alcohol, mean number of drinking days, and relapse rates for up to 12 weeks. The drug appears to be particularly effective in preventing binge drinking among those who relapse.

Leukocytes 4,500/mm³ (4.5 × 10⁹/L)
Platelet count 189,000/mm³
  (189 × 10⁹/L)
Prothrombin time 13 seconds
Hematocrit 34%
Gammaglobulin 1.2 g/dL (12 g/L)
MCV 109 fL (mm³)
Bilirubin 1.3 mg/dL (22.23 µmol/L)
Albumin 3.8 g/dL (38 g/L)
AST 155 U/L
ALT 56 U/L
GGT 190 U/L

Ascitic fluid:
Cell count 200/mm³ (2 × 10⁸/L)
LDH 480 U/L
Glucose 75 mg/dL (4.16 mmol/L)
Bilirubin 0.5 mg/dL (8.55 µmol/L)
Albumin 3.2 g/dL (32 g/L)
Gram stain negative

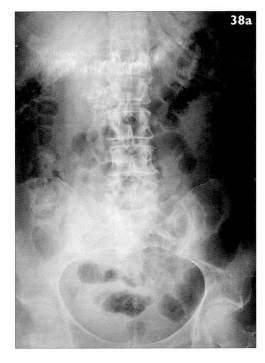

38 A 53-year-old female presents to the emergency room with delusions and extreme agitation. She is an alcoholic. Her family explained that she had been in bed for the previous 3 days unable to take alcohol because of general malaise, nausea and vomiting. Her past medical history was unremarkable apart from her high alcohol intake. On physical examination the patient appeared anxious, shivering, sweaty, and tachycardic. No other neurologic abnormalities were elicited. Her abdomen was distended and a soft and tender liver was palpated. No splenomegaly or chronic liver disease stigmata were noted. Paracentesis revealed a yellowish ascitic fluid. Laboratory investigations are shown.
i. What is revealed by the abdominal X-ray (**38a**)?
ii. Which is the most probable origin of the patient's ascites?
iii. Which other investigations would you undertake?

39 A patient undergoes liver transplantation for cryptogenic cirrhosis. Two days post-operatively, the prothrombin time has increased to 22 seconds and bilirubin and aminotransferase levels are rising. The patient remains comatose and oliguric.
    What is the diagnosis and how is the problem optimally managed?

38 i. The abdominal plain film shows coarse calcification over the pancreatic area, diagnostic of calcific chronic pancreatitis.

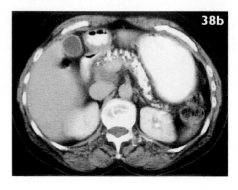

ii. The absence of stigmata of chronic liver disease and laboratory parameters of portal hypertension (namely hypergammaglobulinemia, thrombopenia, and leukopenia) makes the diagnosis of liver cirrhosis unlikely. The presence of a high protein concentration in the ascitic fluid should prompt the search for causes of ascites other than portal hypertension. Once chronic liver disease has been excluded, pancreatic ascites should be highly considered in an alcoholic patient with ascites. Pancreatic ascites occurs insidiously in the setting of chronic pancreatitis, often being the first sign of this disease. It is caused by the leak of fluid from a pancreatic pseudocyst or from the pancreatic duct and is characterized by an increased protein concentration (more than 3 g/dL [30 g/L]) and high levels of amylase (more than 1,000 U/L). This patient had an exudative ascites with amylase of 6,000 U/L.

iii. Apart from the ascitic fluid amylase levels, a CT scan (**38b**) and endoscopic colangiography should be undertaken in order to document the chronic pancreatitis and localize the point of fistulization.

39 This patient exhibits the early signs of primary nonfunction of the liver allograft. In this situation, the liver never functions after transplant and fails to sustain life. Findings include failure of the clinical signs of coagulopathy to correct after reperfusion in the operating room; thereafter, the prothrombin time fails to correct. With a normally functioning graft, the prothrombin time usually begins to correct within a day. Further, in primary nonfunction, the bilirubin will not normalize after transplant. The patient will often not regain normal mental status or renal function and may remain deeply comatose. This is the most reliable indicator of a poor prognosis. In the final stages of liver failure, there are severe alterations of glucose homeostasis with hypoglycemia and hemodynamic instability. Livers that do not function after transplantation must be rapidly replaced if the patient is to survive. A waiting period of >3–7 days is associated with high mortality rates. The causes of primary nonfunction are unknown, but several risk factors have been recognized. The rates of primary nonfunction increase as the cold ischemic time (preservation in chilled solution before transplantation) and the warm ischemic time (the time it takes to implant the liver) increase. Nonfunction is also more common in livers procured from donors requiring pressor support or who had periods of sustained hypotension. Livers with severe macrovesicular steatosis also preserve poorly and exhibit high rates of primary nonfunction. Finally, recipient factors, such as subclinical sepsis, may also contribute to the nonfunction of an otherwise adequate allograft. Unfortunately, these causes of dysfunction are multifactorial, and no preprocurement test accurately predicts the function of a liver following transplantation.

AST 4,200 U/L
ALT 2,860 U/L
Bilirubin 1.2 mg/dL (20.5 μmol/L)
Prothrombin time 16.6 seconds

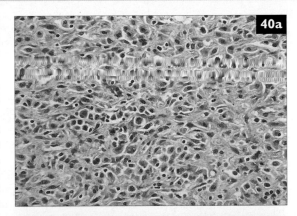

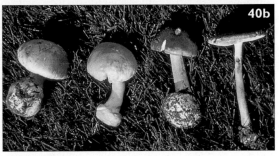

40 A 43-year-old Korean female was admitted to the hospital for abdominal pain, nausea, diarrhea, and mental confusion. There was no past history of liver disease. The patient had recently been hiking in a coastal forest and was known to be a mushroom gatherer. Laboratory investigations are shown. The patient rapidly deteriorated and underwent liver transplantation.

i. Describe the high power histology of the liver (**40a**).

ii. What mushrooms are shown (**40b**)?

iii. What is the diagnosis?

iv. Is there any medical treatment for this condition?

41 A 49-year-old female patient is classified as Child's–Pugh class C on the basis of clinical and laboratory data with a score of 11/15. She has been noncompliant with prior medical therapy and has had two admissions to an alcohol detoxification unit during the last 2 years. The patient presented with a history of hematemesis one day prior to hospitalization and endoscopy revealed large esophageal varices.

What therapy should be undertaken to make recurrent variceal bleeding less likely?

40 i. The high power view of this liver biopsy shows massive hepatic necrosis with no viable hepatocytes identified. There are only residual cellular debris, hemorrhage, and chronic inflammatory cells. In less severe mushroom poisoning, the classic histologic changes consist of zonal necrosis and sinusoidal congestion involving zone 3.

ii. The mushrooms shown in the figure are all *Amanita phalloides*, the death cap, at different stages of maturity. This mushroom characteristically has a ring around the stalk, cup or volva at the bottom of the stalk and white gills. Although not well seen, the mature *Amanita phalloides* often has a distinctive olive green cap. The mushroom to the left is the youngest, probably 3–4 days old, while the mushroom to the far right is the oldest, probably 7–10 days old.

iii. The diagnosis is mushroom poisoning with fulminant hepatic failure. Mushroom poisoning is uncommon in the United States, while several hundred cases are reported on an annual basis in European countries. The amatoxins are the mushroom component primarily responsible for toxicity, with phallotoxins playing a minor role. The clinical features include an acute gastrointestinal phase, followed by a latent phase with few symptoms and a final phase of hepatorenal failure.

iv. Immediately following ingestion, treatment is focused on efforts to prevent absorption, maintenance of fluid and electrolytes and administration of large doses of penicillin. Liver transplantation is life saving in patients who have developed severe hepatic failure.

41 Use of nonselective beta adrenergic blockers (propranolol and nadolol) significantly reduces the risk of recurrent variceal bleeding. The addition of a long acting nitrate such as isosorbide-5-mononitrate produces an incremental reduction in the hepatic venous pressure gradient and may result in a significant decrease in this gradient in patients who were previously characterized as nonresponders to beta blockers. Combination therapy based on reduction in the hepatic venous pressure gradient may significantly increase the efficacy of pharmacologic therapy for the prevention of recurrent variceal bleeding. Although pharmacologic therapy might be an option for a 'more compliant' patient, endoscopic variceal ligation is probably preferable for this patient. The end point of therapy would be the eradication of esophageal varices and the patient should have periodic endoscopic examinations to assess and treat new variceal formation. Variceal ligation is superior to sclerotherapy for reducing the risk of recurrent variceal bleeding, reducing overall mortality and especially mortality related to gastrointestinal bleeding. Ligation is also safer with minimal serious side effects and varices can be eradicated with fewer sessions. Therefore, endoscopic variceal ligation has replaced sclerotherapy as the endoscopic procedure to prevent recurrent variceal bleeding. A meta-analysis of randomized controlled trials comparing the combination of sclerotherapy and propranolol with either sclerotherapy or propranolol given alone shows combination therapy to be efficacious in preventing rebleeding but not in improving survival.

42 A 43-year-old female undergoes liver transplantation for primary biliary cirrhosis. She is treated with antilymphocyte globulin for rejection in the second week and is discharged doing well. Four weeks later she returns with jaundice and complains of mild tenderness of the right upper quadrant. Laboratory data reveal very elevated aminotransferase activities, a slightly elevated WBC count, and eosinophilia. A Duplex sonographic examination (**42a**) shows patent hepatic vessels and no biliary ductal dilation.

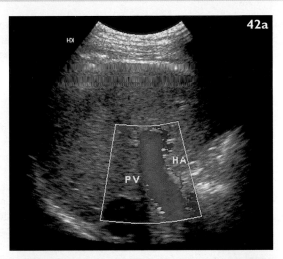

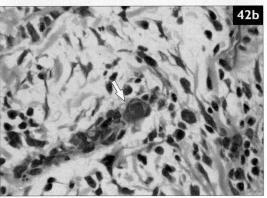

i. Which of the following is the most likely diagnosis:
A Recurrent disease.
B Bile duct stricture.
C CMV infection.
D Acute rejection.

ii. What hallmark histologic findings are shown (**42b**, arrow) and what diagnosis do they confirm?

43 In the process of performing family screening studies on the brother of a well-defined hemochromatosis proband, you find that the brother has a fasting transferrin saturation of 43% and a ferritin of 620 ng/mL (11.09 μmol/L). Genetic studies reveal he a heterozygote for the mutation.
i. What is the significance of his elevated ferritin level?
ii. Will he develop progressive iron-loading?
iii. Should he be treated with therapeutic phlebotomy?

42 i. D. Acute rejection. This patient underwent successful liver transplantation with development of jaundice in the early post-transplant period. Bile duct stricture can cause such a finding but is rarely associated with markedly elevated aminotransferase activities. Stricture is also typically associated with biliary ductal dilation. The cause is usually ischemia. Recurrence of primary biliary cirrhosis after transplantation may occur years after surgery. Both CMV infection and rejection can cause the findings exhibited by this patient. However, the findings of graft tenderness and eosinophilia point to rejection as the cause. Further, viral infections such as CMV are more often associated with a low WBC count and typically occur later in the postoperative period. Other findings associated with CMV infection are pulmonary infiltrates and dyspnea, malaise, and systemic arthralgias. Spiking fevers may be seen in both viral infection and rejection. Rejection is treated with increases in the immunosuppressive regimen, whereas the antiviral agent ganciclovir alone or in combination with intravenous gammaglobulin are the primary treatments for CMV infection.

ii. 42b unexpectedly reveals the typical histologic picture of CMV infection. The most common findings on biopsy in the transplanted liver infected with CMV are a lymphocytic portal infiltrate and focal hepatocyte necrosis with granuloma formation, sometimes referred to as microabscess formation. Intracytoplasmic or intranuclear inclusions are diagnostic and are more common in immunocompromised hosts. Other findings associated with CMV infection are fatty infiltration and Kupffer cell hyperplasia. This patient requires treatment with intravenous antiviral agents. The unexpected histologic findings emphasize the value of liver biopsy in this setting.

43 i. Approximately 25% of heterozygotes for hereditary hemochromatosis have abnormal iron studies. This patient also has mildly abnormal liver enzymes with an ALT of 79 U/L and an AST of 64 U/L. He is about 50 lb (22 kg) overweight. Serological studies, looking for other causes of abnormal liver enzymes, are negative. You suspect that he has nonalcoholic steatohepatitis. A percutaneous liver biopsy is performed that shows moderate degrees of macro- and microvesicular steatosis with an inflammatory infiltrate consistent with the diagnosis of nonalcoholic steatohepatitis. Because the ferritin level was elevated, an hepatic iron concentration is obtained which is 1,400 µg/g with a calculated hepatic iron index of 0.65. His elevated ferritin level is most likely on the basis of nonalcoholic steatohepatitis in the setting of heterozygosity for hemochromatosis. Elevated ferritin levels have been found to be present in about 50% of patients with nonalcoholic steatohepatitis.

ii. Mild iron-loading may occur in heterozygotes, but it is not progressive.

iii. As the iron-loading in hereditary hemochromatosis heterozygotes is not progressive, treatment with therapeutic phlebotomy is not indicated. In patients who have some other type of associated disorder, such as porphyria cutanea tarda along with hereditary hemochromatosis heterozygosity, therapeutic phlebotomy may be beneficial. Therapeutic phlebotomy is not necessary or beneficial in hereditary hemochromatosis heterozygotes.

44 The patient presented with multiple lesions of the extensor surfaces of joints (**44**) .
i. What do these lesions represent?
ii. What is the prognosis of patients with this condition?

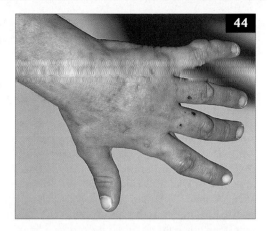

Total serum bilirubin 1.4 mg/dL
    (23.94 µmol/L)
ALT 70 U/L
AST 56 U/L
ALP 240 U/L
GGT 310 U/L.

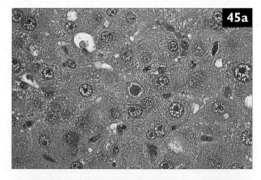

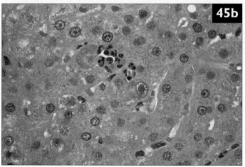

45 A 54-year-old male underwent successful liver transplantation but required OKT-3 for an episode of acute allograft rejection, from which he subsequently recovered. Approximately 7 weeks following transplantation, he noted fatigue, malaise, and low-grade fever. Laboratory investigations are shown. A liver biopsy is performed.
i. What is shown on the liver biopsy (**45a**).
ii. Comment on the liver biopsy findings from a different high power field (**45b**).
iii. What is the diagnosis and what are the clinical features of this infection?
iv. What is the appropriate therapy for this condition?
v. How might this condition best be prevented?

44 i. These are severe cutaneous xanthomas. Serum cholesterol level was approximately 1,000 mg/dL (25.9 mmol/L). The severe cholestasis sometimes observed in Alagille's syndrome is associated with hypercholesterolemia, the deposition of cholesterol in skin, mucous membranes and arteries, and the development of xanthomas. Following liver transplantation, the xanthomas regress slowly over time.
ii. Unfortunately, some cases of Alagille's syndrome have progressed to cirrhosis and development of hepatic malignancy in later years. The management of Alagille's syndrome has been primarily aimed at preventing complications and treating symptoms. Because these patients are cholestatic (reduced bile flow), they are at risk to develop fat soluble vitamin deficiency and have difficulty absorbing fat from their diet. Supplementation of fat soluble vitamins (A, D, E, and K) and monitoring serum levels is warranted in these children in an attempt to maximize their growth and development. In infancy, formulas rich in medium chain triglycerides should be utilized to maximize fat absorption. The itching associated with Alagille's syndrome can be significant and difficult to treat. The use of phenobarbital, cholestyramine, and ursodeoxycholic acid may all be helpful in individual patients. Other drugs (such as antihistamines) may give temporary symptomatic relief. Surgery may on occasion be necessary to obtain an adequate sample of liver tissue to examine the bile duct system. Biliary diversion and Kasai portoenterostomy do not replace bile ducts within the liver and have no value for the patient with Alagille's syndrome. Liver transplantation has been successfully utilized for selected patients with Alagille's syndrome. The associated congenital heart disease may complicate liver transplantation in some of these individuals.

45 i. This liver biopsy shows the classic finding of CMV infection, namely an amphophilic intranuclear inclusion surrounded by a clear halo, such that it resembles an owl's eye. This nuclear inclusion represents closely packed virions.
ii. This biopsy shows focal hepatocyte necrosis with a collection of polymorphonuclear cells, which is another finding characteristic of CMV hepatitis.
iii. The diagnosis is CMV hepatitis. Active CMV infection may result from primary inoculation with the virus or reactivation of latent viral infection. CMV mononucleosis that occurs in immunocompetent adults is a febrile illness with malaise, anorexia, nausea, and vomiting. In immunosuppressed patients, CMV hepatitis with jaundice, pneumonitis, and retinal involvement are all possible complications.
iv. Ganciclovir 5 mg/kg/day is licensed as a specific treatment of CMV-related retinitis in AIDS patients. However, ganciclovir is also routinely used either alone or in combination with CMV immunoglobulin for the treatment of CMV infection in immunosuppressed organ transplant patients.
v. In the setting of organ transplantation, CMV disease is best prevented by intravenous ganciclovir administered early after transplantation when the degree of immunosuppression is high or when additional immunosuppressive therapy is required, such as during treatment of acute allograft rejection with OKT-3 or higher doses of other immunosuppressive agents.

46 A 50-year-old male recently diagnosed with hepatocellular carcinoma presented to an emergency room with confusion and lethargy. He is taking no medications. Neurological examination showed no gross focality and no asterixis.

i. Why is this patient encephalopathic?

ii. What other syndromes can be seen in patients with hepatocellular carcinoma?

47 During a routine physical examination, a 1-year-old female is noted to have a palpable right upper quadrant mass. Her history reveals intermittent episodes of jaundice and abdominal pain reported by her mother.

i. What does the hepatic ultrasound examination reveal (**47a**)? How should one proceed?

ii. Comment on this surgical specimen (**47b**).

iii. What is the likely diagnosis?

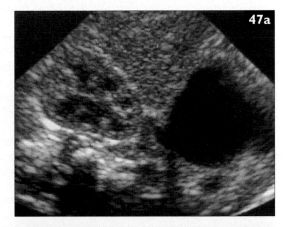

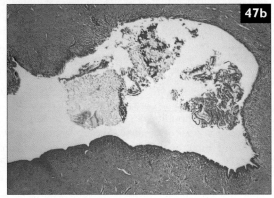

48 On the day of liver biopsy the patient's (see **35**) prothrombin time is 6 seconds prolonged (INR 1.5) and the platelet count is 60,000/mm^3 (60 × 10^9/L).

Which of the following is the most suitable action?

A Continue as planned with no further precautions or therapy.

B Abandon the procedure and initiate immunosuppressive therapy anyway, aiming to undertake biopsy when the biochemical liver tests have improved.

C Use fresh frozen plasma and platelet support to correct the abnormalities and then proceed with the biopsy.

D Recommend transjugular biopsy.

46 i. Encephalopathy in patients with hepatocellular carcinoma is often caused by the underlying cirrhosis and can be treated with lactulose or neomycin. Neoplastic progression in the liver, however, usually results in irreversible hepatorenal failure and encephalopathy. Rarely, hepatocellular carcinoma can disseminate to the brain with subarachnoid or intracerebral hemorrhage from vascular metastases. Occasionally, hepatocellular carcinoma can be associated with paraneoplastic syndromes which simulate hepatic encephalopathy. Hypoglycemia from the secretion of insulin-like growth factors I and II by the hepatocellular carcinoma, and hypercalcemia from tumor production of parathyroid hormone, prostaglandin E, and osteoclast activating factor in the absence of osseous metastases, may cause treatable encephalopathy.

ii. Other paraneoplastic syndromes associated with hepatocellular carcinoma include carcinoid symptoms (ectopic hormone production), erythrocytosis (increased erythropoietin level), hyperthyroxinemia, and porphyria cutanea tarda. These syndromes usually improve with successful treatment of the neoplasm.

47 i. There is a mass within the liver consistent with the findings of a choledochal cyst. This child should have an intraoperative cholangiogram to confirm the diagnosis, define the anatomy of the biliary tree, and to aid in determining the surgical approach.

ii. This specimen is of the cyst wall stained with H&E. It is composed of dense fibrous connective tissue with little muscle or epithelium. Bile is present in the lumen. Residual columnar epithelium is present in the upper left and lower right portions of the slide.

iii. The diagnosis is that of a choledochal cyst. The incidence of choledochal cysts is about 1 in 15,000 live births with girls being affected four times more often than boys. The etiology of choledochal cysts remains uncertain although a congenital defect of bile duct recanalization resulting in a weakness in the bile duct muscular wall is the leading possibility. Bile duct damage may result from reflux of pancreatic enzymes into the common bile duct. Unrecognized choledochal cysts can progress to biliary obstruction and cirrhosis. Excision of the cyst is necessary, if technically feasible, with bile duct anastomosis to the jejunum. It is not acceptable to just aspirate the cyst nor to merely connect the cyst to the jejunum without its removal as there is a risk for the development of adenocarcinoma involving the wall of the cyst. About two thirds of choledochal cysts present before age 10 years. Symptoms as in the present case are often intermittent but progressive and include jaundice, pain, failure to thrive, fevers, and manifestations of a mass. The classic triad of abdominal mass, abdominal pain, and jaundice is seldom present.

48 The optimal requirements for liver biopsy are a prothrombin time <3 seconds prolonged and a platelet count of >100,000/mm^3 (100 × 10^9/L). B, C, and D may all provide reasonable approaches. B is appropriate if the patient is seriously ill and is showing signs of hepatic decompensation, although the prothrombin time will usually be more prolonged as liver failure ensues. A small bleed from the biopsy site may precipitate liver failure. If fresh frozen plasma and platelet transfusion correct clotting abnormalities then the biopsy can be performed. The transjugular approach is appropriate only in very experienced hands – the biopsy specimen is often small.

49 A 57-year-old former alcoholic emphatically claims to be abstinent. Laboratory investigations are shown.
i. What is the significance of the various laboratory test abnormalities?
ii. What means are available to monitor alcohol consumption?

Hemoglobin 14.2 g/dL (142 g/L)
MCV 102.4 fL (mm^3)
Prothrombin time 14.2 seconds
AST 80 U/L
ALT 20 U/L
Albumin 3.8 g/dL (38 g/L)
Total bilirubin 1.2 mg/dL (20.5 µmol/L)
ALP 112 U/L
GGTP 200 U/L

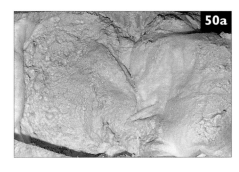
50a

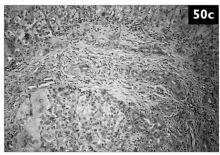
50b

50 A 6-week-old female is brought to the pediatrician by her parents because of concern for unresolving jaundice. Meconium and early stools were normal in color. Laboratory investigations are shown.
i. What is suggested by the appearance of the stools (50a)?
ii. What does this nuclear medicine scan reveal (50b)?
iii. Comment on this percutaneous liver biopsy (50c).
iv. What is the likely diagnosis? What is the treatment?

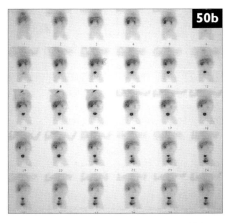
50c

Total bilirubin 6 mg/dL (102.6 µmol/L)
Direct-reacting bilirubin 4 mg/dL (68.4 µmol/L)
AST 200 U/L
ALT 155 U/L

49 i. The MCV, AST, and GGTP levels are frequently elevated in alcoholics.
ii. Self report and physician assessment are unreliable in monitoring sobriety. Indirect laboratory measures, such as elevated MCV, AST, and GGTP levels, are insensitive and nonspecific as they may remain elevated in a large percentage of abstinent patients, especially in those with chronic liver disease. Carbohydrate deficient transferrin results from reduced hepatic glycoprotein glycosyltransferase and increased plasma sialidase activities associated with heavy alcohol consumption, and has been found to be helpful in monitoring alcohol consumption. A commercially available assay for carbohydrate deficient transferrin has high sensitivity and specificity in detecting heavy alcohol consumption (40 g/day), especially in the absence of liver disease. Serial testing can detect relapses before patient self-reporting.

50 i. This stool is white or 'acholic'. This occurs when there is an obstruction to bile flow. Color in stool is dependent upon bile flow and the presence of bilirubin conjugates secreted into the intestinal lumen via the biliary tree. The bilirubin conjugates are converted to pigmented urobilinoids.
ii. This is a hepatobiliary scan demonstrating good uptake of tracer by the liver, but no excretion of isotope into the intestine. Instead, there is excretion of isotope via the kidneys into the urinary bladder. Normally, this technetium labelled isotope when injected into the circulation, is taken up by the liver, and very rapidly secreted into the bile. The isotope will concentrate in the gallbladder and then be excreted, and readily detected in the intestine. If there is bile duct obstruction or diminished bile flow, there will be either a delay or no excretion of the isotope into the intestine. When this occurs, the isotope is cleared via the kidneys and the urinary tract.
iii. This liver biopsy (stained with H&E) displays cholestasis with bile plugs and bilirubinostasis. Note the giant cells and ductular proliferation. There is lymphocytic infiltration in the portal tracts and polymorphonuclear cells between the ductules. Often there is extramedullary hematopoiesis and portal and periportal fibrosis which may progress to cirrhosis if left uncorrected.
iv. The combination of acholic stools, lack of excretion on nuclear medicine scan, and characteristic liver biopsy of ductular proliferation in an infant with a conjugated hyperbilirubinemia is consistent with a diagnosis of biliary atresia. Biliary atresia is estimated to occur in 1 in 8,000 to 1 in 20,000 live births. There is a progressive destruction of the extrahepatic bile ducts during the first months of life. As no single test is diagnostic of biliary atresia, if the initial diagnostic work-up suggests biliary atresia, then an intraoperative cholangiogram to assess patency of the extrahepatic biliary tree is recommended. If extrahepatic biliary atresia is confirmed, then attempted surgical correction with a Kasai portoenterostomy should occur. The Kasai procedure includes excision of the extrahepatic biliary tree in an attempt to identify a ductal remnant at the porta hepatis to which a bowel segment is anastomosed to hopefully re-establish bile flow. Biliary atresia remains the leading cause of pediatric liver transplants in the United States. Early Kasai portoenterostomy may postpone the need for hepatic transplantation until the child is older and larger.

51 A 6-week-old male is seen by his pediatrician for persistent jaundice. The child is breast fed and has pale yellow colored stools. Physical examination reveals a jaundiced infant with hepatomegaly. Laboratory investigations are shown. A

Total bilirubin 6 mg/dL (103 µmol/L)
Direct-reacting bilirubin 4 mg/dL (68.4 µmol/L)
AST 150 U/L
ALT 175 U/L

string test was performed to obtain duodenal bile and reveals yellow pigmented fluid.
What is the differential diagnosis?

52 A 40-year-old female developed a skin abscess and received flucloxacillin 250 mg 4 times daily for 14 days. Past medical history was remarkable for asthma and a 1 week episode of jaundice as a teenager, presumed to have been of viral etiology. Two weeks after completing the antibiotics, she developed malaise, fatigue, pruritus, and jaundice. Serum autoantibodies, viral serology, and other etiological screening tests were negative. Serum levels of ceruloplasmin, alpha-1-antitrypsin, iron, transferrin, and ferritin were normal. An ultrasound examination revealed no evidence of bile duct dilation and an ERCP was normal. The cholestasis persisted, and was unaffected by a 4 week course of prednisone. A percutaneous liver biopsy was obtained at 9 months (52a, immunoperoxidase stain for keratin). Serial biochemical changes are shown (52b).
i. What does the liver histology show?
ii. What is the likely diagnosis?

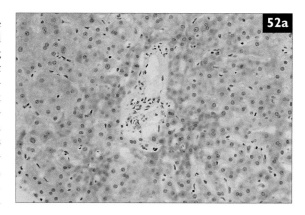

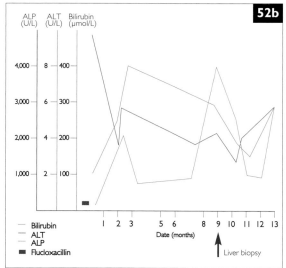

51 The differential diagnosis of conjugated hyperbilirubinemia in an infant is quite long. For simplicity, disorders may be categorized as extrahepatic obstruction, genetic and metabolic disorders, persistent intrahepatic cholestasis, and acquired intrahepatic cholestasis. The term 'infantile obstructive cholangiopathy' has been proposed by Landing to unify the common forms of infantile cholestasis. In neonatal hepatitis, the major involvement is intrahepatic. In biliary atresia, there is progressive fibrosis and ultimate obliteration of the extrahepatic bile ducts. Other causes of biliary obstruction include choledochal cysts, bile plug syndrome, cholelithiasis, spontaneous bile duct perforation, and extrinsic bile duct compression. Genetic and metabolic disorders include disorders of carbohydrate metabolism such as galactosemia, hereditary fructose intolerance, and glycogen storage disease, disorders of amino acid metabolism such as tyrosinemia, and disorders of lipid metabolism such as Niemann–Pick disease, Gaucher disease, Wolman disease, and cholesterol ester storage disease. Chromosomal disorders associated with conjugated hyperbilirubinemia in infants include trisomy 18 and Down's syndrome (trisomy 21). Other genetic and metabolic disorders include alpha-1-antitrypsin deficiency, neonatal hypopituitarism, cystic fibrosis, Zellweger cerebrohepatorenal syndrome, and familial steatohepatitis. Disorders associated with paucity of intrahepatic bile ducts include arteriohepatic dysplasia (Alagille's syndrome), benign recurrent intrahepatic cholestasis, Byler disease, hereditary cholestasis with lymphedema, and hereditary disorders of bile acid synthesis. Acquired intrahepatic cholestasis may be associated with infections such as hepatitis A, B, and C, syphilis, toxoplasmosis, rubella, CMV, herpes, varicella, echovirus, coxsackievirus, leptospirosis, tuberculosis, and bacterial sepsis. Drug induced cholestasis and TPN associated cholestasis may also result in acquired intrahepatic cholestasis.

52 i. A portal tract is shown containing no bile duct. Bile ducts normally show intense staining with the immunoperoxidase stain for keratin. Although slight staining of hepatocytes is evident, no bile duct is seen. The portal vein and artery are present and inflammatory cell infiltrates are absent.
ii. Flucloxacillin-induced cholestasis with a vanishing bile duct syndrome is the likely diagnosis. The prolonged cholestasis observed in this patient can be reasonably ascribed to flucloxacillin for the following reasons: there was no past history of biliary tract disease, and the biliary tract was normal on ultrasonography and on ERCP; there was a close temporal relationship between flucloxacillin administration and the appearance of hepatic dysfunction; other potential causes of vanishing bile duct syndrome such as primary biliary cirrhosis or primary sclerosing cholangitis were excluded on the basis of appropriate serological, histological, and cholangiographic criteria; other drugs able to induce prolonged cholestasis were not taken by the patient at any time before the onset of jaundice.

53 With regard to 52, what is the long term prognosis?

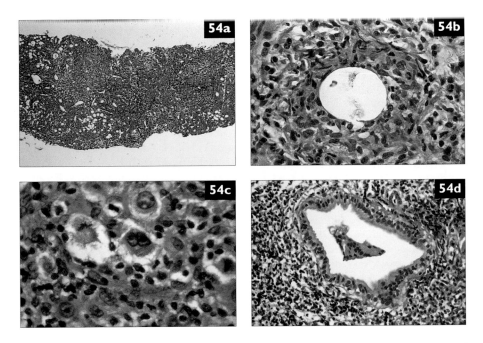

54 A number of chronic liver diseases are characterized by mild, isolated elevation of ALP, or predominant ALP elevation with only slight aminotransferase elevation. All of the liver biopsies shown below came from patients who had isolated or predominant ALP elevation.

i. Describe the biopsy finding (54a).
ii. Describe the biopsy finding (54b).
iii. Describe the biopsy finding (54c).
iv. Describe the biopsy finding (54d).

53 Resolution of symptoms within 6 weeks is the rule, but abnormalities in liver function may persist for months to years in a substantial proportion of patients. Moreover, several patients have developed a syndrome of protracted cholestatic jaundice with progression, in some, to secondary biliary cirrhosis over a period of years. Disappearance of intrahepatic bile ducts occurs in a variety of diseases and congenital conditions, collectively referred to as disappearing or vanishing bile duct syndromes. Drug induced vanishing bile duct syndromes can appear clinically and biochemically similar to primary biliary cirrhosis. This syndrome is characterized by pruritus, hepatomegaly, xanthomas and xanthelasma, and mild steatorrhea. Patients commonly have total bilirubin concentrations above 15 mg/dL (256 μmol/L), persistently elevated serum ALP, hypercholesterolemia, and mildly elevated serum aminotransferase. Liver histology demonstrates canalicular and intracellular cholestasis, but the most striking feature is the paucity of interlobular bile ducts. To date, more than 30 drugs have been reported to induce this syndrome, with chlorpromazine being best documented. Other drugs known to produce these syndromes are similar to chlorpromazine in possessing a polycyclic ring structure. These agents include other phenothiazines, tricyclic antidepressants, haloperidol, and cyproheptadine. Thiabendazole, Augmentin (clavulanic acid/amoxycillin), and flucloxacillin are three other important examples. Liver disease precipitated by flucloxacillin is invariably cholestatic. It may follow a protracted course with the development of vanishing bile duct syndrome. Over 200 cases of cholestatic hepatitis have been reported in association with flucloxacillin. Patients older than 55 and treated for 2 weeks appear to be at highest risk. Although the duration of treatment has varied between a few days to 3 weeks, the onset of symptoms has shown a remarkably consistent delay of 1–3 weeks between cessation of therapy and first manifestations. Patients usually present with jaundice and pruritus. There is marked hyperbilirubinemia and elevation of serum ALP. Aminotransferase levels also are increased, but to a lesser extent. Liver histology typically shows bile stasis with minimal or no hepatitis. Degenerative changes in bile duct epithelium may be marked during the early stages and may progress to depletion of bile ducts, with portal fibrosis and bridging fibrosis. The mechanism of flucloxacillin-induced liver disease is unknown. It appears to represent an idiosyncratic, hypersensitivity phenomenon.

54 i. This biopsy shows micronodular cirrhosis and steatosis, which are suggestive of alcoholic cirrhosis or nonalcoholic steatohepatitis with cirrhosis.
ii. This biopsy shows a granuloma with a clear halo, which is suggestive of Q fever. A distinctive ring pattern in which fibrin is deposited circumferentially within or at the margin of the granuloma may also be seen in some cases.
iii. This biopsy shows atypical histiocytes and classic Reed–Sternberg cells with distortion of normal architecture. This patient had Hodgkin's disease.
iv. This biopsy shows a mixed inflammatory cell and granulomatous infiltrate surrounding an intermediate sized bile duct with hyperplastic bile duct epithelium. This patient had primary biliary cirrhosis.

55 A 46-year-old female presents 5 years after open cholecystectomy. Over this period she has experienced recurrent attacks of typical biliary pain radiating from the right upper quadrant of the abdomen to the back. During these episodes she has been found to have fluctuating abnormal biochemical liver test results, particularly for ALP. Between the attacks the liver tests return to normal. Ultrasound scan shows only a mildly dilated bile duct, a feature commonly seen following cholecystectomy. An ERCP shows no biliary calculi and confirms mild bile duct dilation. Biliary manometry shows a common bile duct pressure of 20 mmHg (2.4 kPa) (normal range up to 10 mmHg [1.4 kPa]). Basal sphincter of Oddi pressure 40 mmHg (5.3 kPa) (normally up to 16 mmHg [2.1 kPa]). Phasic wave amplitude 180 mmHg (24.0 kPa) (normally up to 120 mmHg [16.0 kPa]). Phasic wave frequency is 25/min (normally up to 7/min). An intravenous injection of cholecystokinin precipitated further abdominal pain, increased pressure within the sphincter of Oddi, and increased the frequency of contraction waves.
i. How is the biliary manometry performed?
ii. What are the complications of biliary manometry?
iii. What treatment do you suggest for this patient?

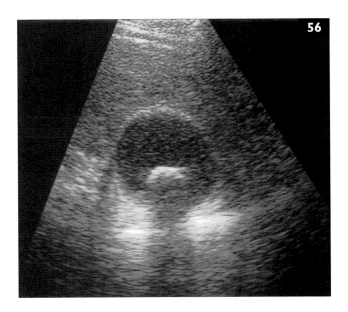

56 A 5-year-old female with cystic fibrosis and pancreatic insufficiency presents to her physician's office with jaundice, right upper quadrant abdominal pain, and fever.
i. What is on this ultrasound scan (56)?
ii. Do the ultrasound findings suggest a likely diagnosis?

55 i. Manometry is performed by introducing a fine catheter deep into the common bile duct and withdrawing it across the sphincter of Oddi. The catheter comprises three pressure ports which are slowly perfused with sterile water. Changes within the perfusion pressures are then displayed and relate to the pressure within the bile duct and sphincter. Cholecystokinin normally reduces both the sphincter of Oddi pressure and the frequency of contraction waves.

ii. The major complication is acute pancreatitis which occurs in up to 10% of patients following manometry.

iii. This patient presents a classic picture of sphincter of Oddi dysmotility. This is characterised by episodic biliary pain following cholecystectomy. Obstruction of the biliary tree causes elevation of ALP concentration and ultrasonic evidence of biliary dilation. At ERCP, drainage of the contrast from the biliary tree may be delayed. It is clearly important to exclude bile duct calculi and an ERCP is mandatory. The manometric findings of raised common bile duct pressure confirm biliary obstruction and this is due to a high pressure tone of the sphincter of Oddi. This patient furthermore displays the abnormality of 'tachy-oddia' in which the frequency of phasic waves is increased. She also displays a paradoxical response to cholecystokinin in which the hormone stimulates rather than relaxes the sphincter. Such a patient requires relief of biliary obstruction by endoscopic biliary sphincterectomy. When a patient presents with a combination of abnormal manometry with a background of abdominal pain and abnormal biochemical liver tests there is an 80% chance of symptoms relief after sphincterotomy. On the other hand if manometry is normal and the only abnormality is that of recurrent biliary pain, it is highly unlikely that sphincterotomy will help.

56 i. This ultrasound scan demonstrates a mobile echogenic, discrete focus within the gallbladder that causes an acoustic shadow. This is most consistent with a gallstone.

ii. The combination of fever, abdominal pain, and jaundice in a patient with a gallstone suggests cholangitis or cholecystitis. Gallstones are a significant clinical problem for children with cystic fibrosis. Estimates of gallstone prevalance range from 12–33% in older children with cystic fibrosis. Cholesterol gallstones in children with cystic fibrosis suggest an imbalance in biliary lipids. Gallstones occur in cystic fibrosis children who also have pancreatic insufficiency suggesting their origin is caused by fat malabsorption or viscous bile due to diminished fluid secretion. Patients with cystic fibrosis and cholelithiasis may be asymptomatic or may present with biliary colic, fever, and jaundice as in the current case. As ultrasonography is noninvasive, it should be considered as the first imaging examination when a child with cystic fibrosis presents with the above symptoms.

57 A 65-year-old male with chronic hepatitis C is referred for evaluation of chronic pruritus. Examination of the skin reveals spider angiomata on the upper thorax and palmar erythema. Laboratory investigations are shown.

Is a normal ALP consistent with the pruritus felt by this patient?

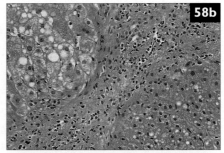

ALP 102 U/L
ALT 166 U/L
AST 205 U/L
Total bilirubin 1 mg/dL (1.11 umol/L)
Direct bilirubin 0.7 mg/dL (11.97 µmol/L)

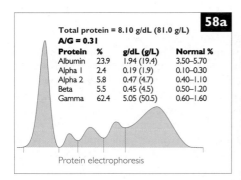

58a

Total protein = 8.10 g/dL (81.0 g/L)
A/G = 0.31

Protein	%	g/dL (g/L)	Normal %
Albumin	23.9	1.94 (19.4)	3.50–5.70
Alpha 1	2.4	0.19 (1.9)	0.10–0.30
Alpha 2	5.8	0.47 (4.7)	0.40–1.10
Beta	5.5	0.45 (4.5)	0.50–1.20
Gamma	62.4	5.05 (50.5)	0.60–1.60

Protein electrophoresis

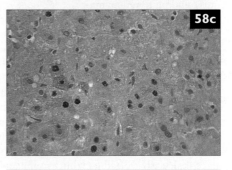

58b

58c

58 A 42-year-old white male was seen because of mild to moderate fatigue, persistently elevated aminotransferase values, and a positive HBsAg test result. He had no risk factors for viral hepatitis. However, his mother died of liver cancer 10 years earlier. He recalls that he had elevated aminotransferase values at the age of 20. Laboratory investigations are shown.
i. Could liver cancer in his mother be a risk factor for hepatitis in this patient?
ii. Comment on the protein electrophoresis results (58a).
iii. Describe the results of a liver biopsy (58b).
iv. Comment on the results of hepatitis B core immunohistologic staining of the liver biopsy (58c).
v. What is the diagnosis and natural history of this condition?

ALT 220 U/L
AST 196 U/L
Platelet count 127,000/mm³ (127 × 10⁹/L)
Bilirubin 0.9 mg/dL (15.4 µmol/L)
Prothrombin time 14 seconds
Alphafetoprotein 3.9 ng/ml
Anti-HCV absent
HBeAg absent
HBsAg present
Anti-HBe present
Hepatitis B virus-DNA 22 pg/mL

57 Yes. Pruritus is one of the common symptoms experienced by patients with cholestatic and other forms of liver disease. Causes of pruritus (i.e. malignancy) not associated with pruritic skin lesions should be considered in patients who present with this symptom. A normal ALP does not rule out liver disease as the underlying cause of pruritus because this symptom does not correlate with serum activity of liver-associated enzymes, levels of serum bilirubin, or bile acids. While bile acids have been implicated in the pathogenesis of this form of pruritus there is no strong scientific evidence that confirms their involvement in this symptom. Clinical studies support the role of endogenous opioids and serotonin in this form of pruritus.

58 i. Yes, if liver cancer in the mother was hepatitis B virus related. Hepatitis B virus could have been transmitted from the infected mother to her offspring either perinatally or during childhood, through intrafamilial contacts.
ii. Protein electrophoresis of the patient's serum shows moderately low albumin and hypergammaglobulinemia. The former is caused by reduced protein synthesis by the liver as a consequence of chronic hepatocellular inflammation and liver parenchyma replacement by fibrosis. The latter reflects polyclonal activation of B cells in response to increased antigen stimulation during portal hypertension.
iii. The liver biopsy shows fibrous expansion and chronic inflammation of the portal areas, central to portal septa and pseudolobular regeneration of hepatic parenchyma. Piecemeal necrosis is present at the interface between portal connective tissue and surrounding parenchyma.
iv. Immunoperoxidase staining of the liver tissue for HBcAg, showing staining of liver cell cytoplasm and nuclei. In patients infected with precore/core mutants of hepatitis B virus, HBcAg is also localized in the liver cell cytoplasm. Infection with wild strains of hepatitis B virus more often shows HBcAg in the liver cell nuclei than infection with mutant strains.
v. Chronic infection with precore 'mutant' strains of hepatitis B virus leading to chronic active hepatitis and cirrhosis. The diagnosis is based upon low titer serum hepatitis B virus-DNA coexisting with anti-HBe. In 'wild' type hepatitis B, high titer serum hepatitis B virus-DNA coexists with serum HBeAg. Patients with hepatitis B virus related cirrhosis are at risk of clinical decompensation with jaundice, ascites, encephalopathy, bleeding from esophageal varices, and hepatocellular carcinoma. The annual rate of hepatocellular carcinoma development is 3–6%, but it may be higher in patients with elevated serum levels of alphafetoprotein.

59 With regard to 58:
i. What further investigations are indicated?
ii. What treatment is indicated?

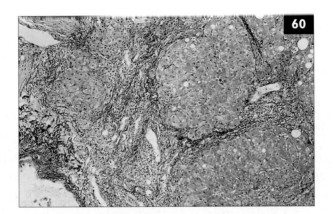

60 A 56-year-old carpenter was referred for evaluation of abnormal liver test results and a positive hepatitis C antibody test. Twenty-two years earlier he had received 3 units of blood to treat hematemesis caused by a duodenal ulcer. Three weeks later he developed jaundice and elevated serum ALT values. Physical examination showed mild hepatomegaly. Spleen span was 11 cm (4.3 in). Laboratory investigations are shown. Ultrasound examination shows mild to moderate liver enlargement.

ALT 120 U/L
AST 87 U/L
Platelet count 16,000/mm³ (16 × 10⁹/L)
Albumin 3.2 g/dL (32 g/L)
Prothrombin time 13.5 seconds
Anti-HBc present
Anti-HBs present
Anti-HCV present
Ferritin 600 ng/mL (12.0 µmol/L)

i. Describe the liver biopsy results (60).
ii. What is the diagnosis and natural history of the disease?
iii. What further investigations are indicated?

61 A 2-month-old male is seen for routine pediatric care and noted to be jaundiced. On physical examination, there is hepatomegaly. Family history is significant for emphysema in his paternal grandfather at an early age. Laboratory investigations are

Total bilirubin 6 mg/dL (102.6 µmol/L)
Direct-reacting bilirubin 4.5 mg/dL (77 µmol/L)
AST 150 U/L
ALT 149 U/L

shown. Inadvertently, a serum protein electrophoresis was ordered and revealed a diminished alpha-1-globulin peak.
What laboratory tests would you order to confirm the diagnosis?

59 i. This patient would require upper gastrointestinal endoscopy to define the presence of esophageal varices, regular monitoring with abdominal ultrasounds, and laboratory examinations including alphafetoprotein. Family contacts should be investigated for markers of hepatitis B virus and susceptible individuals vaccinated against hepatitis B virus.
ii. Persistent liver cell inflammation related to virus replication may lead to hepatic decompensation or hepatocellular carcinoma; thus, antiviral treatment is an option. Interferon-alpha may suppress virus replication and attenuate liver cell inflammation in 20–40% of these patients. Lamivudine or other antivirals may also suppress viral replication and improve liver injury.

60 i. The liver biopsy shows mononuclear infiltrates of portal tracts with fibrosis and bridging septa. There is cirrhosis with nodular regeneration of the parenchyma. Piecemeal periportal necrosis and macrosteatosis is present (Masson stain).
ii. Transfusion-associated chronic hepatitis C virus infection leading to active cirrhosis. Hepatitis C infection has been a common sequela to blood transfusion, however, following implementation of screening programs of donors, this mode of transmission of hepatitis C has been virtually eliminated. Transfusion associated hepatitis C infection becomes chronic in approximately 70–80% of cases, and 20% of them may develop cirrhosis. The time lag between infection and cirrhosis may be 20–30 years, but it may be as short as 3 years in immunocompromised patients. hepatitis C virus related cirrhosis usually is a long lasting, slowly progressive disease with an expected, 10 year survival rate of 75%. Clinical decompensation, rupture of esophageal varices and hepatocellular carcinoma are common causes of death.
iii. This patient would require assessment for tissue autoantibodies, thyroid stimulating hormone, alphafetoprotein, and upper gastrointestinal endoscopy. Sexual contacts should be investigated for the presence of serum hepatitis C antibodies.

61 Diagnosis is confirmed by determining the alpha-1-antitrypsin phenotype. Serum alpha-1-antitrypsin levels may be useful but on occasion may be misleading as they may increase in response to inflammation. As 90% of the alpha-1-globulin peak on serum protein electrophoresis is due to alpha-1-antitrypsin, a diminished or absent alpha-1-globulin peak on serum protein electrophoresis may be a useful screening tool. The alleles of the principal gene coding for alpha-1-antitrypsin are collectively known as the protease inhibitor (Pi) system. The allele products (Pi phenotypes) are designated by letters corresponding to the electrophoretic mobility of the protein. The normal allele is designated PiM (medium fast). Abnormal alleles associated with liver disease include PiS (slow) and PiZ (ultra slow). Homozygous PiZZ has been classically associated with liver disease. Curiously, not all patients with PiZZ phenotype develop liver or lung disease in spite of low alpha-1-antitrypsin levels.

62 A 38-year-old male sewage worker notices that his urine has become unusually dark, and subsequently develops mild malaise, right upper quadrant discomfort, and jaundice.

i. What is the diagnosis?

ii. What groups of people are most at risk from this disease?

iii. Briefly discuss its epidemiology.

63 A 45-year-old female with an unremarkable past medical history presents with progressive abdominal distension. On examination, evidence of ascites and tender hepatomegaly are noted. No stigmata of chronic liver disease are seen. The patient's complaints started 2 months earlier. She denies taking oral contraceptives or any other drugs and there are no risk factors for viral hepatitis. Laboratory investigations are shown.

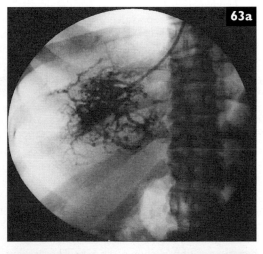

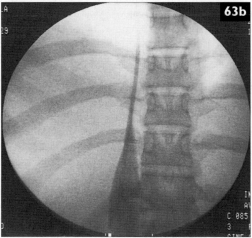

i. What is revealed on the hepatic venography (**63a**) and the photograph of the inferior vena cava (**63b**)?

ii. What is the etiology of this condition?

iii. Which are the potential therapies?

AST 59 U/L
ALT 73 U/L
ALP 378 U/L
GGT 63 U/L
WBC count 6,100/mm³
    (6.1×10^9/L)
Platelet count 180,000/mm³
    (180×10^9/L)
Prothrombin time 14 seconds
Ascitic fluid protein 5 g/dL (50 g/L)
Ascitic cell count 400/mm³ (4×10^8/L)
    (predominantly mononuclear)

62 i. The most likely diagnosis is hepatitis A, although Weil's disease (from *Leptospira icterohaemorrhagiae* or *canicola*) should be considered. Weil's disease is characterised by severe myalgias and renal failure.

ii. Anyone exposed to raw sewage; travellers to underdeveloped countries, particularly in rural areas; and offenders and staff in penal institutions, drug users, and homosexual men are all at increased risk. Patients and health care staff, especially those involved in the care of the mentally ill or handicapped, and staff looking after nontoilet trained children are also at risk.

iii. The hepatitis A virus has a worldwide distribution, with very high seroprevalence in Africa, high seroprevalence in Amazonian Brazil, intermediate in Mediterranean Europe, low in the USA, and very low in Scandinavia. Within these areas, however, there is a wide variation in seroprevalence, usually dependent upon socioeconomic status. In countries with very low endemicity, hepatitis A virus occurs almost exclusively in adults returning from areas of high endemicity, or in drug users. In areas of very high anti-HAV seroprevalence, 90% of children are infected by 5 years of age, whereas in areas of high endemicity there is a lower prevalence in 5 year olds, but 90% prevalence is reached in 10 year olds. In intermediate areas, this degree of prevalence is only reached by young adulthood, and in areas of low prevalence there is a gradual rise from 15% at 15 years to 75% at 50 years. As countries develop, and living conditions and sanitation improve, hepatitis A virus prevalence rates fall dramatically. There is a safe and effective vaccine for hepatitis A.

63 i. Following hepatic vein injection of contrast medium, numerous hepatic venous collaterals are shown (**63a**) giving the classic spider web appearance of the Budd–Chiari syndrome. Marked narrowing of the inferior vena cava in its retro-hepatic position is shown on **63b**. This is caused by the caudate lobe hypertrophy typical of this condition.

ii. Budd–Chiari syndrome includes a variety of pathologic processes which obstruct the progression of blood from the liver into the right atrium. Conditions that affect the hepatic venules are commonly referred to as hepatic veno-occlusive diseases, and are most commonly seen following the administration of cytotoxic agents or radiation therapy. Occlusion of the major hepatic veins (as in this patient), is usually related to an underlying hypercoagulable state such as myeloproliferative disorders, systemic lupus erythematosus, paroxysmal nocturnal hemoglobinuria, antithrombin III deficiency, protein C deficiency, oral contraceptive use, or the postpartum period. Budd–Chiari syndrome can also be the result of obstruction of the inferior vena cava (due to a membranous intracaval web or caval thickening).

iii. The mainstay of therapy has traditionally been surgical intervention, particularly portosystemic shunting and liver transplantation. However, the recent appearance of the TIPS represents a unique therapy that can, if technically possible to perform, actually undo the pathologic process. Although long term follow-up is lacking, if feasible this option seems to be the best therapy. If the presence of cirrhosis is established with certainty, however, most clinicians would favor transplantation.

64 A 52-year-old male with a 20 year history of chronic alcoholism presents with increasing jaundice of 1 month duration. Physical examination reveals profound icterus, spider angiomata, tender hepatomegaly, and asterixis. The laboratory results at admission and after 1 week are shown. Percutaneous liver biopsy is illustrated (64a, b).

i. What considerations are in the differential diagnosis of the patient's jaundice?
ii. Which diagnostic tests are indicated?
iii. What abnormality is shown in the liver biopsy?
iv. What is this patient's prognosis?
v. How should this patient be treated?

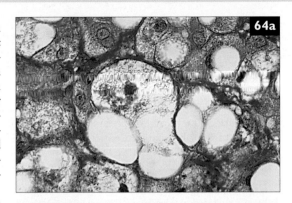

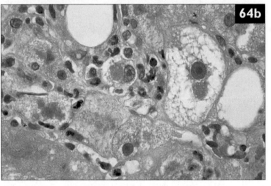

	Admission	1 week
AST	219 U/L	25 U/L
ALT	32 U/L	34 U/L
ALP	386 U/L	27 U/L
GGTP	416 U/L	324 U/L
Total bilirubin	17.4 mg/dL (297 µmol/L)	21.4 mg/dL (366 µmol/L)
Albumin	3.0 g/dL (30 g/L)	2.9 g/dL (29 g/L)
Prothrombin time	16.0 seconds	18.7 seconds

65 A 28-year-old male medical resident is working the night shift in a busy county hospital. One of his colleagues notices that his sclerae are icteric and tells him. He says that he has Gilbert's syndrome.
i. What is the cause of hyperbilirubinemia in Gilbert's syndrome?
ii. What is the expected serum bilirubin level in this man?

64 i. Hepatitis (alcoholic, viral, drug) should be considered in the differential diagnosis, as should biliary obstruction (elevated ALP and GGTP).
ii. Viral serologies for hepatitis viruses A, B, and C and abdominal ultrasound.
iii. The biopsy reveals the classic findings of alcoholic hepatitis. **64a** shows hepatocyte ballooning and degeneration, steatosis, and pericellular fibrosis. In **64b** polymoropho-nuclear leukocyte infiltration is present.
iv. The clinical manifestations of alcoholic hepatitis are highly variable. Severe episodes are characterized by prolonged (months) and progressive hepatic failure with mortality rates of hospitalized patients as high as 65%. In a retrospective analysis of patients, findings associated with early death included presence of hepatic encephalopathy, degree of bilirubin elevation, and prothrombin time prolongation. A discriminant function formula (DF) to predict survival follows:

$$DF = 4.6 \text{ (prothrombin time} - \text{control prothrombin time)} + \text{serum bilirubin (mg/dL)}$$

A DF score above 32 identifies the patients at risk of early mortality (50% risk of death within 2 months).
v. Most patients with alcoholic hepatitis have evidence of nutrient depletion as a result of inadequate intake, calorie displacement by alcohol, and the inflammatory state. A high calorie, high protein nutritional supplement has been shown to improve hepatic function and reduce mortality in patients at risk for early death from moderate to severe alcoholic hepatitis without exacerbating hepatic encephalopathy. Mortality is reduced by corticosteroids in severe disease without gastrointestinal hemorrhage or infection. In general, patients should be observed for 5–7 days after hospitalization before beginning treatment. Prednisolone is recommended (40 mg/day for 4 weeks, then a 2 week taper). Pentoxifylline, an inhibitor of tumor necrosis factor alpha, has been shown to improve short-term survival and decrease the risk of developing the hepatorenal syndrome.

65 i. Defective glucuronidation of bilirubin caused by decreased activity of hepatic bilirubin uridine diphosphate-glucuronyltransferase.
ii. Unconjugated hyperbilirubinemia of about 3 mg/dL (51.3 μmol/L). Gilbert's syndrome is a benign condition that occurs in approximately 5% of the general population; it is more common in males. The syndrome is characterized by uncon-jugated hyperbilirubinemia of modest degree which can be exacerbated by fasting or low calorie intake, intercurrent illnesses, and stress. The criteria for the diagnosis of Gilbert's syndrome are asymptomatic unconjugated hyperbilirubinemia in individuals with no abnormalities in any of the liver-associated enzyme activities or bile acids, no evidence of hemolysis, and no stigmata of liver disease. The pathogenesis of Gilbert's syndrome is not completely understood. There is impaired glucuronidation of bilirubin. This defect was recently reported to be, in part, caused by mutations in the 5' promoter region of the gene that codes for bilirubin uridine diphosphate-glucuronyltransferase 1, the enzyme responsible for most of the glucuronidation of bilirubin. The mutation is characterized by homozygosity for two extra bases (TA). In addition to a glucuronidation defect, studies of bromosulphothalein and indocyanine green clearance suggest abnormalities in bilirubin uptake.

66 A 24-year-old Italian, male drug addict has a rapid onset of fatigue and jaundice. Laboratory investigations are shown.
i. What is the diagnosis?
ii. Could a liver biopsy be safely performed and, if yes, would it be necessary to confirm the diagnosis?
iii. Which kind of treatment would you suggest?
iv. What is his short and long term prognosis?

AST 2.6 U/L
ALT 4.9 U/L
Prothrombin time 25 seconds
Albumin 3.7 g/dL (37 g/l)
Hemoglobin 14.5 g/dL (145 g/L)
WBC count 9,400/mm³ (9.4 × 10⁹/L)
Platelet count 158,000/mm³ (158 × 10⁹/L)
HBsAg present, IgM anti-HBc absent, HBeAg present, hepatitis B virus-DNA present
Anti-HD present, IgM anti-HD present
Anti-HCV absent

AST 64 U/L
ALT 86 U/L
ALP 294 U/L
GGT 1,254 U/L
Serum bilirubin normal
Albumin normal

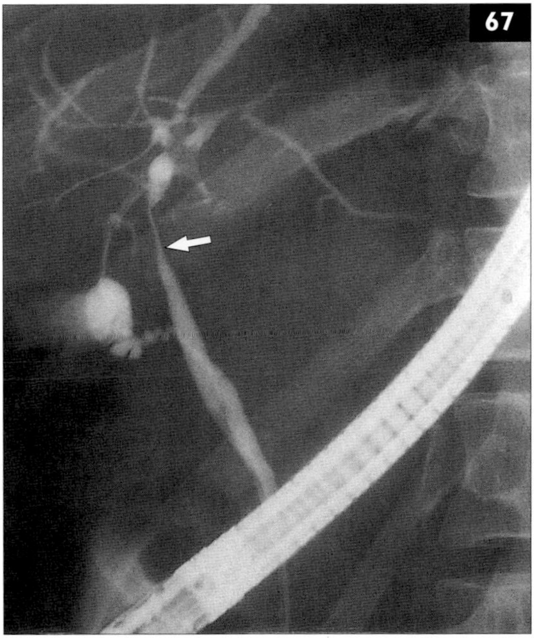

67 A 37-year-old male photographer was found to have an elevated ALT at the time of blood donation. He was asymptomatic and a later physical examination was normal. There was no history of alcohol use or risk factors for viral hepatitis. Laboratory investigations are shown. Ultrasound examination of the abdomen was normal.
i. What is revealed by the pattern of liver test result abnormalities?
ii. What does the cholangiogram (67, arrow) show? What is the diagnosis?

66 i. The diagnosis is acute hepatitis related to hepatitis D virus superinfection of a patient chronically infected by hepatitis B virus. The diagnosis of superinfection is supported by the presence of high titers of IgM anti-HD and the lack of serum IgM anti-HBc. If the patient had not been already infected by hepatitis B virus and had been coinfected by hepatitis B and D viruses at the same time, both IgM anti-HBc and IgM anti-HD would have been present at the onset of the disease. The absence of detectable anti-HCV at the time of acute hepatitis does not rule out a possible coinfection with hepatitis C virus. The patient must be tested again for anti-HCV 3 months after the acute episode or for hepatitis C virus-RNA immediately.
ii. Due to the prolonged prothrombin time a liver biopsy cannot be safely performed. The diagnosis of acute hepatitis caused by hepatitis D can be easily made on the basis of the biochemical and serological pattern and does not require any further histological support. A liver biopsy performed during the acute phase of hepatitis D virus superinfection would not help to stage the underlying chronic hepatitis B.
iii. The only therapeutic option for hepatitis D is interferon, but there is no evidence that its administration during the acute phase of hepatitis D virus disease could be of any benefit. The patient has to be carefully monitored in order to discover any sign suggesting a progression to fulminant hepatitis. Superinfection with hepatitis D virus of a chronic carrier of hepatitis B virus bears a high risk of fulminant hepatitis.
iv. If the patient survives the acute episode of hepatitis, the risk of developing chronic hepatitis D is up to 90%, sustained, as in this case, by persistent replication of hepatitis B virus. Hepatitis D virus chronic hepatitis can rapidly evolve to cirrhosis and liver failure; otherwise if active replication of both viruses subsides the disease can enter an indolent phase characterized by reduced biochemical and histological activity, still progressing to liver failure within 20 years from the acute infection.

67 i. The nearly threefold elevation of ALP, 15-fold elevation of GGT with twofold elevation of aminotransferase activities represents a cholestatic biochemical liver test result profile. This pattern of liver enzyme activity elevation is compatible with chronic cholestatic liver diseases, such as primary biliary cirrhosis or primary sclerosing cholangitis, or extrahepatic biliary tract obstruction from conditions such as cholelithiasis or carcinoma of the pancreas. In other noncholestatic liver diseases such as chronic viral hepatitis, aminotransferase elevation is more characteristic of hepatocellular injury; serum aminotransferase activities are elevated variably from slightly increased to 10-fold, while ALP is almost double.
ii. The cholangiogram shows a prominent stricture of the common hepatic duct immediately below the confluence of the right and left hepatic ducts. The intrahepatic ducts, although poorly filled, show beading and irregularity. These findings are compatible with primary sclerosing cholangitis. This diagnosis is characterized by a cholestatic biochemical profile and the above cholangiographic findings. Liver biopsy typically shows portal tract inflammation and periductal fibrosis. Survival time to liver transplantation approximates 12–15 years after diagnosis.

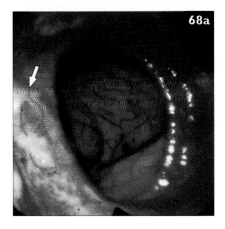

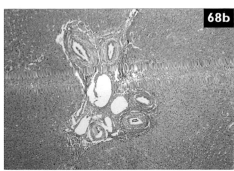

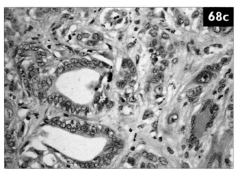

68 i. With regard to the case in **67**, comment on the subsequent sigmoido-scopic findings (**68a**, arrow).
ii. Comment on the findings of this wedge liver biopsy obtained 6 weeks after initial diagnosis (**68b**).
iii. What is revealed on the liver biopsy obtained 10 years following the original diagnosis (**68c**).
iv. What medical or surgical therapy is appropriate?

69 A 52-year-old male is referred for evaluation of abnormal liver tests. He has been drinking 6–8 beers/day for many years. However, he has previously been able to stop completely for up to 6 months without difficulty, and his alcohol use has never adversely affected his personal or professional life. As a result of a liver biopsy which reveals significant septal fibrosis, he decides to lead a more healthy lifestyle. He has stopped smoking, lost 15 lb (6.8 kg), and reduced his alcohol consumption to at most 2 beers/day. He states that a friend told him that colchicine is good for the liver and asks for advice concerning a variety of nutritional supplements which he purchased at his local health food store, including 'extra strength' multivitamin tablets with iron, folic acid, selenium, beta carotene, vitamin A, and vitamin C.
i. Which vitamin deficiencies are present in alcoholic liver disease?
ii. Which supplements are potentially hepatotoxic in this patient?
iii. What is the pathophysiology of their interactions with alcohol?

68 i. Sigmoidoscopic findings show erythema, ulceration, and exudate involving the rectosigmoid mucosa in a diffuse pattern characteristic of ulcerative colitis. Approximately two thirds of patients with primary sclerosing cholangitis have inflammatory bowel disease; 85–90% have ulcerative colitis, and the rest have Crohn's colitis. Inflammatory bowel disease is often diagnosed several years earlier than primary sclerosing cholangitis. Ulcerative colitis can, however, be diagnosed simultaneously with primary sclerosing cholangitis or years later.
ii. This low power view of the liver biopsy shows striking periductal fibrosis.
iii. This biopsy shows histologic changes compatible with cholangiocarcinoma, which may develop during the course of primary sclerosing cholangitis in 10–15% of patients. Patients who appear to be at highest risk for cholangiocarcinoma are those with cirrhosis on liver biopsy and long standing ulcerative colitis. This biopsy shows gross distortion of the bile duct epithelium, which is dysplastic and disorganized.
iv. There is no medical therapy proven to delay progression of primary sclerosing cholangitis. Short term studies showed improvement of liver enzymes with ursodeoxycholic acid administration, but long term prognosis is unknown. Endoscopic therapy is appropriate for patients who have a dominant stricture amenable to balloon dilation. Indications for endoscopic therapy are jaundice or recurrent bacterial cholangitis. Biliary diversion therapy, popular in the past, is less often performed with the demonstrated effectiveness of endoscopic therapy. Patients with end-stage secondary biliary cirrhosis are candidates for liver transplantation. In general, transplantation should be performed somewhat earlier in the course of end-stage liver disease because of the risk of cholangiocarcinoma.

69 i. Nutritional deficiencies are common in alcoholic liver disease. Hepatic vitamin A levels, in particular, are strikingly depressed, even in the absence of obvious dietary deficiency and in those with only a fatty liver in whom serum vitamin A and prealbumin levels are normal. Experimentally, chronic ethanol consumption speeds hepatic vitamin A degradation. Similarly, retinol and retinoic acid breakdown is accelerated by the induction of microsomal enzymes caused by chronic ethanol consumption. In addition, the conversion of carotenoids to retinoids is impaired. Other deficiencies commonly associated with alcoholic liver disease involve thiamine, folate, ascorbic acid, selenium, and alpha-tocopherol (vitamin E).
ii. Vitamin A, beta carotene, and iron may be toxic to the liver. Iron potentiates experimental ethanol toxicity by increasing lipid peroxidation. Supplemental iron therapy should be limited to those patients with a documented deficiency and promptly discontinued when iron levels are restored.
iii. Although hepatic vitamin A deficiency is usually present in patients with alcoholic liver disease, caution should be stressed regarding replacement therapy because interactions with ethanol can increase toxicity. For example, plasma beta carotene levels are increased by even moderate alcohol consumption. In experimental animals beta carotene supplements produce an increased inflammatory response and more prominent degenerative cellular changes in the liver. In addition, hepatic fibrosis can directly result from high doses of vitamin A.

70 A 25-year-old HIV positive female was hospitalized with abdominal pain, nausea, myalgias, and malaise of 10 weeks duration. Her medications included zidovudine 200 mg three time daily, fluconazole 100 mg four times a day, and ranitidine 150 mg twice daily. Physical examination revealed an ill-appearing, obese young woman

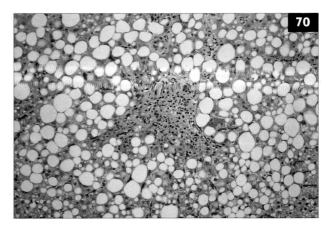

weighing 200 lb (91 kg). Her heart rate was 124 beats/min and blood pressure 95/70 mmHg (12.7/9.3 kPa). The sclerae were anicteric and there were no stigmata of chronic liver disease. Abdominal examination revealed hepatomegaly (vertical span 15 cm [5.8 in]). The laboratory results and results of serological testing for viral hepatitis are shown. An abdominal ultrasound examination demonstrated mild splenomegaly and diffuse gallbladder wall thickening without cholelithiasis or dilation of the biliary tree. A percutaneous liver biopsy was performed (70).
i. Comment on liver biopsy histology.
ii. What is the etiology of this clinical condition?
iii. What is the pathogenesis of this condition?

AST 759 U/L
ALT 459 U/L
ALP 182 U/L
Total bilirubin 1.8 mg/dL (30.8 µmol/L)
Prothrombin time 12 seconds
CD4 lymphocyte count 460/µL
Sodium 140 mEq/L (140 mmol/L)
Chloride 108 mEq/L (108 mmol/L)
Bicarbonate 12 mEq/L (12 mmol/L)
Creatinine 0.8 mg/dL (70.7 µmol/L)
Amylase 380 U/L
Creatine phosphokinase 3450 U/L

Anti-HBc IgG present
HBsAg absent
Anti-HCV absent

71 In patients with documented portal vein obstruction, complications related to extra-hepatic portal hypertension may occur. Children with cavernous transformation of the portal vein benefit from a functionally normal liver and the potential to develop collateral varices which may result in decompression of the portal system.

What therapy should be considered for children presenting with variceal bleeding as a consequence of cavernous transformation of the portal vein?

70 i. The biopsy shows macrovesicular steatosis or large droplet fatty change. The portal zone contains minimal inflammatory cells.

ii. Zidovudine (AZT) induced hepatic steatosis associated with severe lactic acidosis (anion-gap metabolic acidosis). Attention has focused recently on a syndrome of marked hepatic steatosis associated with severe lactic acidosis. In some patients treated with nucleoside analogs for HIV infection and also hepatitis B this progressed to hepatic failure.

iii. The mechanism of nucleoside induced hepatic steatosis and lactic acidosis is not understood, but considerable evidence points towards disruption of mitochondrial DNA and failure of mitochondrial oxidative metabolism. This results in the accumulation of fat in hepatocytes, failure of lactate metabolism, depletion of ATP, and subsequent profound failure of hepatocellular function. Accompanying multisystem abnormalities such as the pancreatitis and myopathy evident in this patient may reflect disruption of mitochondrial function in a variety of tissues by AZT. Similar syndromes have been described in patients treated with didanosine and in patients with hepatitis B treated with the experimental drug fialuridine (FIAU). The syndrome of hepatomegaly with steatosis has been described in several patients receiving AZT. This association has been striking enough to prompt a letter to physicians from the manufacturer in June 1993 and a boxed warning in the AZT label. Most cases of this syndrome have been reported in female patients. This suggests that there may be a gender-related predisposition to this particular toxic effect, and that the failure to detect this type of toxicity in early trials may have reflected their overwhelming preponderance of male subjects. Affected patients have commonly been obese with the onset of symptoms after at least 6 months of treatment. Patients have typically presented with nonspecific gastrointestinal complaints and hepatomegaly, and the majority have developed profound lactic acidosis with several fatalities. Biochemical liver test abnormalities have been notable for moderate elevation of aminotransferase activities with minimal or no increases in serum ALP and bilirubin levels. Hepatic histology showed severe macrovesicular steatosis with minimal necrosis or inflammation.

71 Extrahepatic portal vein obstruction is associated potentially but infrequently with life threatening gastrointestinal hemorrhage. The time from obstruction to hemorrhage can be very variable, if ever. The lack of significant liver disease as opposed to intrahepatic portal hypertension makes extrahepatic portal hypertension more benign. Treatment must be tailored to each patient. As many children with extrahepatic portal vein thrombosis will 'outgrow' their portal hypertension as a result of recanalization and development of collaterals, observation and minimally invasive procedures are recommended. Variceal bleeding is the most dramatic and potentially life threatening complication. Variceal bleeding should be treated with sclerotherapy or band ligation in anticipation of the patient 'outgrowing' the problem. Other treatment modalities such as surgical shunting, transjugular intrahepatic portosystemic shunts, or splenic embolization used in children with intrahepatic causes of portal hypertension with bleeding, should be reserved for patients unresponsive to endoscopic therapy.

72 An 82-year-old male amputee presents to hospital with rigors, jaundice, and abdominal pain. Abdominal ultrasound suggests that the intrahepatic biliary tree is dilated and following resuscitation, he was referred for an ERCP.
i. What abnormalities are seen on the ERCP (72)?
ii. What treatment is indicated?

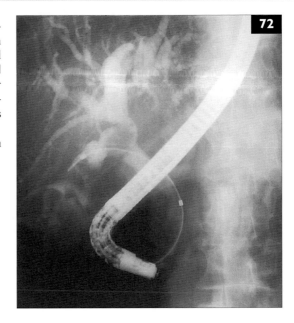

73 A previously healthy 13-year-old female presents with rapid (over 1 month) onset of jaundice, increasing abdominal girth, and obtundation. She is jaundiced, has ascites, hepatosplenomegaly, and mild hepatic encephalopathy. She has taken no medication but a family history reveals a maternal grandparent who died of liver disease at age 35. She was inoculated with hepatitis B vaccine 3 years ago. An ultrasound examination of the liver showed no evidence of biliary obstruction or hepatosplenomegaly. Laboratory investigations are shown.
i. What diagnosis should be considered?
ii. What specific examinations and tests should be obtained?
iii. What treatment should be initiated?

Hemoglobin 8.4 g/dL (84 g/L)
Platelet count 50,000/mm³ (50 × 10⁹/L)
Prothrombin time >20 seconds
ALT 180 U/L
AST 250 U/L
Albumin 1.8 g/dL (18 g/L)
ALP 160 U/L
Bilirubin, total 10.2 mg/dL (174.4 µmol/L)
    direct bilirubin 5.0 mg/dL (85.5 µmol/L)
Coombs test negative
Heterophile negative
HBsAb present

72 i. The ERCP shows that there is considerable dilation of the intrahepatic biliary tree associated with a stricture within the common hepatic duct. The ERCP cannula passes from the biliary tree straight into the gallbladder which is packed with stones. The stricture is caused by compression of the biliary tree by the stones within the gallbladder. The combination of extrinsic compression of the common bile duct by calculi with fistulation between the bile duct and the gallbladder is known as Mirizze's syndrome. This syndrome is unusual and may alternatively be caused by gallbladder cancer. It is thought that compression of the biliary tree by the stone in Hartmann's pouch or the cystic duct leads to ulceration and fistulation. The fistula usually communicates with the common bile duct although communication with the intrahepatic biliary tree is also described.

ii. The initial priority is to relieve obstructive jaundice. Biliary obstruction is not caused by common bile duct stones and sphincterotomy is necessary. A plastic biliary stent is inserted via the endoscope in order to drain the bile duct. This may be difficult because the guidewires involved in placing the stents tend to pass directly into the gallbladder via the fistula rather than into the common hepatic duct. If endoscopic stenting proves impossible, percutaneous radiological stenting is indicated. Following relief of jaundice and alleviation of sepsis the patient requires an open cholecystectomy and hepaticojejunostomy. More conservative forms of therapy are associated with bile duct stricturing.

73 i. The possible etiologies of rapidly progressive hepatic failure include toxic ingestions, viral hepatitis, autoimmune hepatitis, Reye's syndrome, and the fulminant presentation of Wilson's disease should be considered. A family history of liver disease should alert one to the possibility of an inherited metabolic disorder. The presence of a Coombs negative hemolytic anemia and liver disease is highly suspicious for the fulminant form of Wilsonian liver disease.

ii. A slit-lamp examination for Kayser–Fleischer rings should be obtained, but may not be positive in a young patient with Wilson's disease. Serum ceruloplasmin activity is reduced in 90% of patients with Wilson's disease. In the hemolytic phase of Wilson's disease, both serum copper concentration and urinary copper content are markedly elevated. For uncertain reasons, the serum ALP activity is only minimally increased in proportion to the increase in serum bilirubin in fulminant Wilsonian hepatitis even when the rise in bilirubin caused by hemolysis is accounted for. When the diagnosis of Wilson's disease is established, all other siblings should be screened for this disorder.

iii. Patients presenting with fulminant hepatitis caused by Wilson's disease should be given chelational therapy with penicillamine. However, at this stage of the disease most progress to hepatic failure and death despite pharmacologic therapy. These patients should, therefore, be referred to centers which perform liver transplantation. Patients with fulminant Wilson's disease who have undergone hepatic transplantation have survival rates of nearly 90%. Following hepatic transplantation patients no longer require treatment for Wilson's disease as this procedure provides a phenotypic cure.

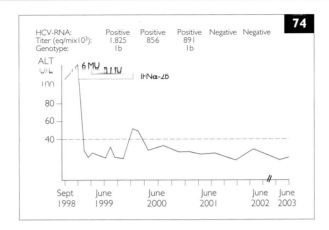

HCV-RNA:	Positive	Positive	Positive	Negative	Negative
Titer (eq/mix10³):	1,825	856	891		
Genotype:	1b		1b		

74 i. How should patients with chronic hepatitis C and chronic hepatitis on biopsy be treated?
ii. Can patients achieve long term absence of hepatitis C virus-RNA in serum and normal aminotransferase values following anti-viral therapy?
iii. What factors may help predict response to therapy?
iv. This graph (**74**) indicates this patient's response to interferon. Comment on the follow-up of this patient.

	Day 1	Day 3	Day 6
AST	8,200 U/L	1,000 U/L	400 U/L
ALT	4,100 U/L	800 U/L	200 U/L
ALP	200 U/L	180 U/L	
GGTP	280 U/L	260 U/L	
Total bilirubin	4.0 mg/dL	8.2 mg/dL	2.4 mg/dL
	(68.4 μmol/L)	(140.2 μmol/L)	(41 μmol/L)
Prothrombin time	14 seconds	16 seconds	12.8 seconds

75 A 50-year-old chronic alcoholic presents with jaundice after taking an unclear number of acetaminophen tablets for a headache following a binge. Physical examination reveals asterixis. Laboratory investigations at admission and over the next week are shown.
i. What is the etiology of the patient's jaundice?
ii. What additional diagnostic tests are indicated?
iii. How are the liver tests, and especially the serial examinations, helpful in determining the etiology of this patient's jaundice?
iv. How does chronic alcohol abuse contribute to the liver damage present in this patient?

74 i. Liver cell inflammation relating to persistently replicating hepatitis C virus is responsible for the progression of the disease. To stop hepatic inflammation pegylated interferon administered weekly in combination with ribavirin administered twice daily can be used for a maximum of 12 months. Thirty to 50% of patients infected by genotype 1 and 60–80% of those infected by genotype 2 or 3 of HCV will have sustained disease remission and permanent virus eradication. The ideal treatment duration is 6 months for genotype 2 or 3 patients, whereas treatment should be extended to 12 months for genotype 1 patients who show a virological response at months 3–6 of treatment. Interferon plus ribavirin therapy is more likely to be successful in young patients, those with a low pre-treatment viremia, those without cirrhosis, and alcohol abstainers. Females and normal body weight persons are also more likely to respond to treatment.

ii. Yes. Normal serum ALT/AST, and a negative serum hepatitis C virus-RNA by PCR assay in the years following interferon cessation suggest long term cure in up to 20% of all treated patients. Patients who remain serum hepatitis C virus-RNA positive even though they have persistently normal ALT/AST are at great risk of hepatitis recurrence. Treatment success is even more impressive with interferon–ribavirin therapy, particularly in infections with hepatitis C virus of genotypes other than type 1.

iii. Although liver histology and virus genotype and load may predict response to interferon, no absolute indicator of response has been defined. There are at least 6 different genotypes of hepatitis C virus. In Japan, Europe, and the US, infections with genotype 1 are most common and show greater resistance to interferon therapy than genotypes 2 or 3. Patients with chronic hepatitis C have wide ranges of serum hepatitis C virus-RNA levels, from <50 IU/L up to millions IU/L. Patients with <800,000 IU/L have responded better to interferon than those with higher levels of viremia.

iv. The graph shows early ALT response to interferon treatment, followed by persistent ALT normalization after treatment cessation. The interesting finding is delayed clearance of serum hepatitis C virus-RNA, which became undetectable by PCR only 1 year after treatment cessation. Delayed loss or failure to lose hepatitis C virus-RNA may indicate a higher chance of disease recurrence after therapy has been discontinued.

75 i. Acetaminophen toxicity exacerbated by chronic alcoholism is most likely.

ii. Serological tests for hepatitis A, B, and C are indicated.

iii. Alcoholic patients with acetaminophen hepatotoxicity often present with mild to moderate jaundice, coagulopathy, and abnormal aminotransferase levels with an AST to ALT ratio >1. Peak aminotransferase activities are usually present on admission, and levels rapidly decline over several days. In alcoholic hepatitis aminotransferase levels are only modestly elevated, and values are usually <300 U/L. Although extreme aminotransferase elevation is unusual for viral hepatitis, acute infectious hepatitis should always be considered, and serologic testing is indicated.

iv. Usually acetaminophen is metabolized to nontoxic glucuronic acid or sulfate conjugates which are then excreted by the kidneys. Hepatic mixed-function oxidase activity metabolizes a small fraction of the dose to reactivate electrophilic glutathione conjugation. As chronic alcohol consumption increases production of toxic metabolites while simultaneously depleting glutathione, potentially fatal hepatotoxicity can result from even moderate therapeutic doses (2.4–4 g).

76 A 36-year-old, white male presents for evaluation of abnormal liver enzymes and elevated iron studies. He has a remote history of intravenous drug abuse but now works as an attorney. Laboratory studies show a normal CBC, an ALT of 110 U/L, an AST of 86 U/L, with normal bilirubin, albumin, and ALP. A nonfasting transferrin saturation is slightly increased at 55%. The serum ferritin is 650 ng/mL (11.6 µmol/L). An anti-HCV by ELISA is present.

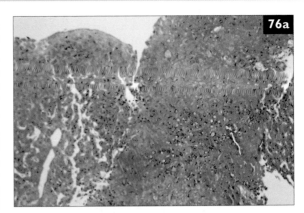

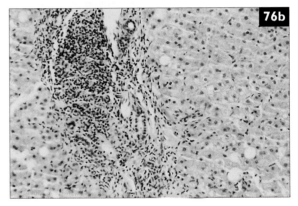

i. What is the most likely cause of this individual's abnormal iron studies?
ii. A liver biopsy was performed (76a, b). What is the indication for this procedure?

77 A 69-year-old female is referred for evaluation of fatigue and abnormal liver biochemical profile. Investigation of her liver disease led to the diagnosis of cirrhosis due to alpha-1-antitrypsin deficiency. Selected laboratory investigations are shown.

What is the nature of the prolonged prothrombin time in this patient?

ALP 308 U/L
ALT 38 U/L
AST 90 U/L
Total bilirubin 1.9 mg/dL (32.5 µmol/L)
Albumin 0.25 g/dL (2.5 g/L)
Prothrombin time 15 seconds
Platelet count 84,000/mm³ (84 × 10⁹/L)

76 i. It is likely that this patient has abnormal iron studies in association with chronic hepatitis C. About 40–50% of patients with chronic viral hepatitis, alcoholic liver disease, and nonalcoholic steatohepatitis have abnormal iron studies and do not have hemochromatosis. Usually, these abnormal iron studies are limited to an elevated serum ferritin level with a normal or only slightly increased transferrin saturation. In this patient, the transferrin saturation was obtained in a nonfasting state and as many as 50% of individuals will have 'falsely' elevated transferrin saturations when drawn in this fashion. When looking for hemochromatosis, blood studies of iron metabolism should be obtained in the morning in the fasting state. The reason for the increased ferritin level is most likely due to its being an acute phase reactant and, or, its being released from tissue iron stores because of hepatocellular necrosis.

ii. Before the discovery of the hemochromatosis gene, HFE, the only way that patients with homozygous hereditary hemochromatosis could be accurately distinguished from patients with liver enzyme abnormalities associated with necroinflammatory liver disease, hereditary hemochromatosis heterozygotes, or from patients with liver disease and mild secondary iron overload, was to perform a percutaneous liver biopsy both for histochemical iron stains and for biochemical determination of hepatic iron concentration. A liver biopsy would be performed on this patient to define the extent of injury from HCV and assess the amount of tissue iron by histopathological examination including Perls' Prussian blue stain and for hepatic iron concentration. From the hepatic iron concentration, the hepatic iron index could be calculated. Currently, HFE mutation analysis for C282Y and H63D would be performed. C282Y homozygosity is found in approximately 90% of patients with typical hemochromatosis. Studies of C282Y heterozygosity in patients with chronic hepatitis C have shown no increase in prevalence over that of the general population. However, in C282Y heterozygotes who have chronic hepatitis C, the hepatic iron concentration is slightly increased and the development of fibrosis is enhanced. With HFE mutation analysis, the use of hepatic iron index is less important in determining which patients have hereditary hemochromatosis. In recent studies, as many as 15% of patients who are C282Y homozygotes have hepatic iron indexes <1.9, but virtually all of them have elevated hepatic iron concentrations.

77 Liver function is impaired in this patient as reflected by her low albumin levels and prolonged prothrombin time. One of the functions of the liver is the production of coagulation factors (fibrinogen, prothrombin, and factors V, VII, IX, X, and XII) with the exception of von Willebrand factor and fibrolytic proteins. It also produces inhibitors of coagulation such as protein C and antithrombin III. As the liver fails, the production of these factors decreases.

78 With regard to the patient in 77:
i. What is the predicted response of this patient to vitamin K therapy?
ii. What is the etiology of her thrombocytopenia?

79 A 23-year-old male presented with anorexia and nausea, epigastric pain, light stools, dark urine, pruritus, and weight loss. His pattern of liver test abnormalities and diagnostic tests are shown on **79a.**
i. Describe the CT findings (**79b**).
ii. Describe the findings on percutaneous transhepatic cholangiography (**79c**).
iii. Describe the liver biopsy findings (**79d**).
iv. What is the diagnosis?
v. What clinical and pathologic features characterize this unusual variant?

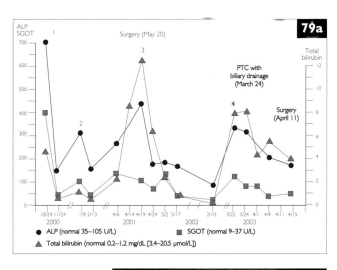

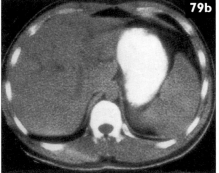

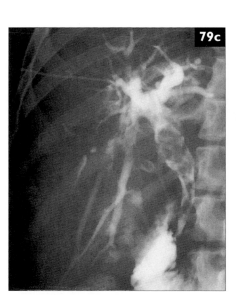

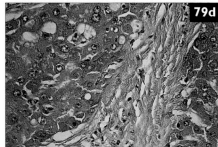

78 i. The coagulopathy of patients with advanced liver disease is caused by decreased production of clotting factors. Vitamin K is necessary for production of coagulation factors. A component of the coagulopathy may be caused by malabsorption of vitamin K due to cholestasis and, therefore, the coagulopathy may respond to some degree to vitamin K administration. However, the coagulopathy is not completely corrected by administration of this vitamin. In general, a therapeutic trial of subcutaneous vitamin K for 3 days is administered to correct a potential vitamin deficiency, but beyond that, supplementation of this vitamin is not recommended because it is not helpful.

ii. Thrombocytopenia occurs in approximately 30% of patients with cirrhosis and is as common as 50% in patients with decompensated liver disease. The pathogenesis of thrombocytopenia is multifactorial. Factors underlying increased platelet destruction include: increased platelet pooling in the spleen which does not correlate with spleen size, decreased platelet half-life, disseminated intravascular coagulation, and immune-mediated platelet destruction. Factors contributing to decreased production include: bone marrow suppression caused by nutritional deficiencies (e.g. folic acid) and thrombopoietin deficiency. Thrombopoietin is a recently characterized protein which contributes to platelet formation. It is produced primarily by the liver but also by the bone marrow, kidney, and spleen. Thrombopoietin is not normally detected in the serum, however, it becomes measurable in conditions associated with thrombocytopenia (e.g. chemotherapy). Patients with cirrhosis and thrombocytopenia, however, do not produce measurable concentrations of thrombopoietin.

79 i. This CT scan shows dilated intrahepatic bile ducts.

ii. This percutaneous cholangiogram shows a dilated bile duct with intraductal filling defects.

iii. This biopsy shows large polygonal tumor cells separated by lamellae of fibrous tissue.

iv. The diagnosis is fibrolamellar carcinoma of the liver. The tumor grew into the biliary tract and caused intermittent bile duct obstruction.

v. Fibrolamellar carcinoma differs from the ordinary hepatocellular carcinoma in that there is no underlying viral cirrhosis and the mean age of onset is younger, often in adolescence. Over 90% of fibrolamellar carcinomas occur in patients younger than 25. The tumor is also more slowly growing and has a better prognosis, including after liver transplantation which is associated with a 40–50% 5 year survival versus 20–40% survival for the usual hepatocellular carcinoma.

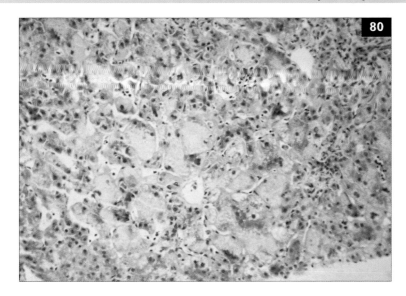

80 A 6-week-old child undergoes a thorough evaluation for conjugated hyper-bilirubinemia. A liver biopsy is performed as part of this investigation (**80**).
i. What should the thorough evaluation entail?
ii. Does the liver biopsy suggest a diagnosis?

81 An exploratory paracentesis is per-formed on a 65-year-old cirrhotic patient with ascites who presents with transient fever and vague abdominal complaints. The results of laboratory investigations on ascitic fluid obtained is shown. Due to the spontaneous disappearance of fever and the normality of ascitic fluid and

Ascites fluid:
Protein 1.5 g/dL (15 g/L)
WBC count 400/mm³ (4 × 10⁸/L)
(90% mononuclear cells)
Glucose 70 mg/dL (3.88 mmol/L)
LDH 120 U/L

WBC count no antibiotics are given. The patient is discharged. However, 2 days later *Escherichia coli* grows on the ascitic fluid culture.
i. Would you consider this an episode of spontaneous bacterial peritonitis?
ii. Should antibiotics have been prescribed from the beginning?
iii. Would you undertake further examinations? Should antibiotics be prescribed at this time?

80 i. The major goals of the evaluation are to identify those infants with treatable infectious and metabolic disorders, recognizable genetic or congenital disorders, or extrahepatic obstruction who would benefit from surgical therapy. A complete physical examination and medical history are essential. Ophthalmologic examination by an experienced ophthalmologist may demonstrate cataracts, retinopathy, or optic nerve hypoplasia. The laboratory evaluation begins with fractionation of serum bilirubin. For conjugated hyperbilirubinemia, the evaluation proceeds with determination of serum aminotransferase activities, ALP activity, albumin, cholesterol, and a prothrombin time. Examination of a fresh stool specimen for pigment color is cheap and very useful. White or acholic stools demand a speedy evaluation to determine the cause as surgical correction of biliary atresia is time dependent. The best results are obtained if surgery is performed before 2 months of age. Cultures, viral titers, immunoglobulin levels, VDRL, viral hepatitis serologies, and bone radiographs may suggest infectious disorders. A sweat chloride test or genetic marker screen may suggest cystic fibrosis. The presence of a low alpha-1-antitrypsin level should be followed by protease inhibitor (Pi) typing to establish a diagnosis of alpha-1-antitrypsin deficiency. An abdominal ultrasound examination may reveal a choledochal cyst, abdominal mass, biliary stone, ascites, and presence or absence of the gallbladder. A string test to obtain duodenal bile for pigment color is a simple and useful procedure. Hepatobiliary scintigraphy, after several days of phenobarbital therapy to stimulate bile flow, may help to distinguish impaired uptake of isotope from the inability to excrete isotope because of biliary obstruction.
ii. Liver biopsies from an infant with neonatal hepatitis usually demonstrate a marked infiltrate of inflammatory cells in the portal area, focal hepatocellular necrosis, giant cell transformation, extramedullary hematopoiesis, and bile stasis. In contrast to biliary atresia, there is no evidence of bile duct proliferation in this specimen. This slide shows the prominent giant cell transformation (H&E). The findings in this case are consistent with idiopathic neonatal hepatitis. Therapy is directed at maintaining adequate fat and fat soluble vitamins using vitamins and medium chain triglyceride supplements. Drugs used to stimulate bile flow might include phenobarbital, cholestyramine, and ursodeoxycholic acid. Prognosis is variable and dependent upon the degree of residual fibrosis, but most patients usually resolve their jaundice and do well.

81 i. Spontaneous bacterial peritonitis is excluded because the criterion of >250 poly-morphonuclear leukocytes/mm³ (2.5 × 10⁸/L) in ascitic fluid is not fulfilled.
ii. Neither the medical history nor the initial laboratory investigations indicate a diagnosis of bacterial peritonitis, hence no antibiotics should have been prescribed.
iii. It is important to repeat the paracentesis in these cases. Spontaneous bacterial peritonitis is diagnosed if more than 250/mm³ (2.5 × 10⁸/L) polymorphonuclear leukocytes are detected. On the other hand, if no changes are noted in the ascitic fluid, the episode is named bacterioascites; in this setting no antibiotics need be given. Bacterioascites is defined as the passage of bacteria from the bloodstream to ascites without the development of a true infection (due to a high opsonic activity of ascitic fluid or to a small septic load).

AST 98 U/L
ALT 90 U/L
ALP 200 U/L
GGTP 280 U/L
Total bilirubin 1.2 mg/dL
   (20.5 μmol/L)
Prothrombin time
   12.8 seconds

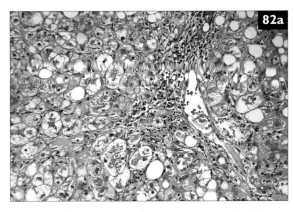

82 A 40-year-old male with a remote history of intravenous drug use is referred for evaluation of abnormal biochemical liver tests associated with positive hepatitis C virus serology. He currently drinks six beers daily. Laboratory investigations are shown. Percutaneous liver biopsy is illustrated (**82a, b**).

i. Comment on the pattern of the liver test results.

ii. Comment on the liver biopsy.

iii. What is the role of viral hepatitis in alcoholic liver disease?

iv. What are the treatment options for this patient?

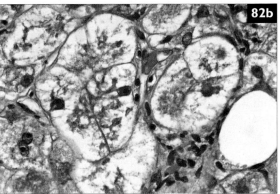

83 A healthy 5-year-old male whose older sibling was recently diagnosed at age 12 as having Wilson's disease was referred by his physician for evaluation. Both parents are in good health. His physical examination is normal. Slit-lamp examination showed no Kayser–Fleischer rings visible. His ultrasound examination showed a normal liver. His liver biopsy had normal histology. Laboratory investigations are shown.

Hemoglobin 13 g/dL (130 g/L)
Platelet count 175,000/mm³ (175 × 10⁹/L)
ALT 20 U/L
AST 55 U/L
Ceruloplasmin 15 mg/dL (150 mg/L)
Quantitative 90 μg/g dry weight hepatic copper

What further testing should be performed? Is treatment necessary?

82 i. AST and ALT are elevated to the same degree. In alcoholic liver disease (without coexisting viral infection), the AST is usually significantly greater than ALT (ratio usually >2), and in viral hepatitis the ALT is most often greater than the AST.

ii. Evidence of both viral (periportal fibrosis, portal lymphoid infiltration, and interface hepatitis in **82a**) and alcoholic injury (ballooning degeneration in **82b**) is present. Steatosis is commonly seen in both alcoholic liver disease and infection with hepatitis C.

iii. The presence of portal and, or, lobular inflammation is strongly associated with chronic hepatitis C infection in alcoholic patients. Hepatitis C infects between 24–54% of alcoholic patients undergoing liver biopsy. Alcohol consumption may accelerate the liver disease caused by hepatitis C infection. Viral hepatitis may also account for the occasional patient in whom there is histologic progression of liver disease despite abstinence from alcohol.

iv. Abstinence is the cornerstone of therapy. Treatment of the actively drinking patient using pegylated interferon-alpha with ribavirin is not recommended as these patients are frequently noncompliant and both alcoholism and interferon therapy produce similar adverse hematologic effects (neutropenia and thrombocytopenia). In addition, efficacy is reduced. However, such therapy can be considered in the abstinent patient in whom liver biopsy reveals pathologic injury consistent with active viral infection. Vaccination for hepatitis B should be considered for all patients without evidence of previous exposure. Although the response to the standard vaccine dose is suboptimal in patients with chronic alcoholism, an increased dose as is recommended for hemodialysis patients (40 µg at 0, 1, 2, and 6 months) is effective.

83 Wilson's disease is inherited in an autosomal recessive fashion. The normal health of the parents suggest that they are both heterozygous for the Wilson's disease mutation. The likelihood of this patient having Wilson's disease is therefore 25%, of being a heterozygote 50%, of being unaffected 25%. The reduced level of serum ceruloplasmin suggests that this sibling of a patient with Wilson's disease is either a patient or a carrier of the gene for Wilson's disease. The lack of Kayser–Fleischer rings in this young patient does not exclude Wilson's disease as these are often seen with increasing age in untreated patients. The normal hepatic histology and copper level of 90 µg/g dry weight indicates that he does not have Wilson's disease but is a carrier. Most normal individuals have hepatic copper levels that are 40 µg/g dry weight liver or less. The intermediate levels of hepatic copper seen in many heterozygotes are not pathologic and these patients will not develop the hepatocellular injury associated with the elevated levels of hepatic copper in patients with Wilson's disease. No treatment is necessary.

84 A 60-year-old white male was first noted to have abnormal biochemical liver test results on routine monitoring after 18 months of amiodarone treatment. His liver span measured 16 cm (6.2 in) in the right midclavicular line; the edge was easily palpable and was firm and nontender. He had palmer erythema, but no spleno-megaly or ascites. Amiodarone was discontinued and a liver biopsy was performed (84a, b). The patient admitted to heavy alcohol ingestion in his youth but had been abstinent from alcohol for the past 22 years. He had no past clinical or labora-tory evidence of liver disease.

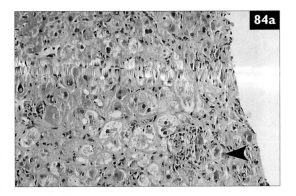

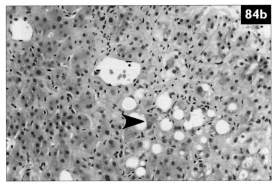

i. Comment on the liver his-tology, in particular the areas indicated by the arrows (84a, b).
ii. What is the most likely diag-nosis?
iii. What other histological findings may be present?
iv. What is the management and long term outcome of this clinical condition?

AST 520 U/L
ALT 131 U/L
Bilirubin 1.0 mg/dL (17.1 μmol/L)
ALP 229 U/L
Prothrombin time 11.4 seconds
Albumin 3.9 g/dL (39 g/L)

85 One month later the patient in **35** and **48** is asymptomatic and the biochemical liver tests have returned to the normal range on 15 mg prednisolone/day.
i. Should the next step be to withdraw all treatment and follow-up at 3 month intervals or, alternatively, add azathioprine (1 mg/kg) and after 1 month, gradually reduce the dose of prednisolone to 10 mg/day over the next 2 months?
ii. What are the acute side-effects of azathioprine and what precautions should be taken to avoid them?

84 i. 84a shows mild fibrosis, hepatocyte swelling with focal cytoplasmic accumulation of Mallory hyaline (arrow), and a mild inflammatory reaction (consisting of polymorphonuclear cells). 84b shows the centrilobular zone with macrovesicular fat and Mallory hyaline (arrow).

ii. Amiodarone induced nonalcoholic steatohepatitis. Alcohol as a component is unlikely given discontinuation of alcohol intake 22 years before treatment and that his baseline biochemical liver tests were normal.

iii. On electron microscopy, the liver biopsies from patients treated with amiodarone reveal a striking accumulation of concentric, whorled membranous arrays (myeloid figures) in lysosomes, similar to those seen in hereditary lipidoses such as Niemann–Pick and Tay–Sachs diseases. Amiodarone accumulates in hepatic lysosomes and induces the formation of these structures, which represent phospholipids but appear to play no role in the development of toxicity.

iv. Amiodarone should be discontinued when liver enzymes increase above two times the upper limit of normal. A liver biopsy should be considered to aid in the diagnosis. Amiodarone induced liver abnormalities usually resolve slowly over several weeks to months after withdrawal. Owing to slow release of the drug from storage deposits, hepatic abnormalities may persist for up to 1 year after discontinuation, and liver disease may even worsen. Mild hepatotoxicity is common with amiodarone therapy. The most frequent finding is asymptomatic elevation of serum aminotransferase activities (up to fivefold) in approximately 40% of patients receiving long term therapy. In some patients values have returned to normal during continued treatment. The most common clinical finding is hepatomegaly; jaundice is unusual. Liver biopsy in cases of severe toxicity typically shows features similar to those in alcoholic hepatitis, such as steatosis, focal necrosis, focal (predominantly polymorphonuclear) leukocyte infiltrates, centrizonal fibrosis, and perinuclear (Mallory's) hyaline inclusions. Also, liver biopsy almost always shows phospholipids. The histologic appearances of cholangitis may be present, and granulomas have been observed. In several cases, the liver lesion has progressed to a micronodular cirrhosis, with death sometimes ensuing. Acute injury may also occur with amiodarone. There have been several reports of acute hepatotoxicity within hours to days after intravenous loading of the drug. The acute injury is believed to be immunoallergic, but whether this is caused by amiodarone itself or by an organic surfactant (polysorbate 80) added to intravenous amiodarone formulations is unclear.

85 i. The correct course would be to add azathioprine. The minimum duration of treatment is 2 years. Several years are usually required. Severe relapses occur after early withdrawal of treatment (or too rapid a reduction) and may be fatal within 3 months of withdrawal. Introduction of azathioprine allows the steroid dose to be decreased.

ii. Lethargy and headaches necessitating drug withdrawal occur in about 10% of cases. Myelosuppression is the major side-effect and CBCs should be monitored. Note, however, that low WBC counts and thrombocytopenia may be attributable to concomitant hypersplenism so that it is a fall in the counts, rather than the absolute count, that are an indication for withdrawal. (See also **129**.)

86 A 54-year-old female underwent hepatic transplantation because of liver failure resulting from end-stage primary biliary cirrhosis. The operation was arduous because of extensive varices but after 7 hours the procedure was completed. Immunosuppression was started immediately using a combination of prednisolone, cyclosporin, and azathioprine. Initial renal dysfunction rapidly resolved and over the first few days she made good progress. On the 7th day she developed fever and increasing jaundice.

i. What is the diagnosis at this point?

ii. A diagnostic test was undertaken. What examination is this (86)?

iii. What abnormality is demonstrated?

iv. What treatment is required?

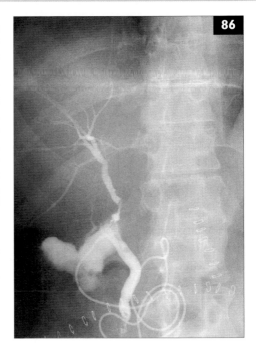

87 A 60-year-old male cirrhotic patient with ascites presented with a 1 year history of exertional dyspnea. The patient had a positive serology for hepatitis C virus and had been diagnosed with cirrhosis 7 years previously, after a first episode of ascites. He was able to control his ascites with a low-sodium diet and moderate doses of diuretics. He had suffered two episodes of hepatic encephalopathy. On examination the patient was slightly tachypneic (18 breaths/min), and clubbing, moderate ascites, and small bilateral pleural effusions were noted. Laboratory investigations are shown.

Hemoglobin 11 g/dL (110 g/L)
Platelet count 110,000/mm^3
   (110 × 10^9/L)
Bilirubin 2.5 mg/dL (42.75 μmol/L)
Prothrombin time 21 seconds
Albumin 2.8 g/dL (28 g/L)
Sodium 128 mEq/L (128 mmol/L)
Potassium 4.3 mEq/L (4.3 mmol/L)
Total lung capacity 82%
PaO_2 59 mmHg (7.9 kPa)
$PaCO_2$ 32 mmHg (4.3 kPa)
DL_{CO} 30%
FEV_1 80%

i. What do the arterial blood gases and the pulmonary function test indicate?

ii. What is the most likely diagnosis?

iii. What further investigations should be undertaken?

iv. Which is the best treatment for this patient?

86 i. The differential diagnosis includes graft rejection, ischemia, sepsis, and biliary disease. Acute rejection is found in up to 30% of patients following hepatic transplantation and occurs between the 4th–14th day postoperatively. Patients present with malaise, abnormal biochemical liver test results, and tender enlargement of the liver. Liver biopsies are diagnostic. Ischemia resulting from hepatic artery thrombosis usually occurs at an early stage following an operation. It is associated with rapid failure of the liver graft with severe cholestasis. Sepsis is a strong possibility in view of the long arduous operation in a presumably malnourished and immunosuppressed patient. Biliary pathology is possible either from a leak at the anastomosis of the biliary tree or an ischemic stricture.

ii. The test is a T-tube cholangiogram. Hepatic transplantation involves primary anastomosis between donor and recipient biliary tree and a gallbladder conduit is no longer used.

iii. The T-tube cholangiogram shows contrast leaking from the biliary anastomosis.

iv. The treatment of choice is operative bile duct repair. In particularly ill patients, a biliary stent can be introduced endoscopically or percutaneously as a temporary measure but this may be technically demanding and risks introduction of infection.

87 i. The arterial blood gases show substantial hypoxemia, which is even greater when the rapid respiratory rate is considered. The high alveolar–arterial oxygen gradient of 61 mmHg (8.1 kPa) together with the decreased DL_{CO} reflect a profound impairment of gas transfer. Lung volumes are normal.

ii. Several derangements of pulmonary function have been described in patients with cirrhosis including a restrictive pattern of lung function, air flow obstruction, and an increased alveolar–arterial oxygen gradient. Moreover, pleural effusions and decreased lung volumes caused by tense ascites frequently lead to dyspnea. However, the profound hypoxemia seen in this patient, together with clubbing and severely increased alveolar-arterial oxygen gradient point to the hepatopulmonary syndrome.

iii. With reference to arterial blood gases, 80–90% of patients with hepatopulmonary syndrome develop platypnea and orthodeoxia, defined as the development of shortness of breath and reduction in PaO_2, respectively, when moving from the supine to the standing position. This phenomenon is caused by an increased blood flow through vascular dilations in the lung bases. Although not specific, in the setting of liver disease, this is virtually diagnostic of hepatopulmonary syndrome. The most sensitive diagnostic test for detecting these intrapulmonary vascular dilations, however, is contrast-enhanced echocardiography.

iv. To date, medical therapy of hepatopulmonary syndrome has been disappointing. Recent reports have documented reversibility of hepatopulmonary syndrome after liver transplantation. In this patient, in whom the coexistence of hyponatremia and severe hepatocellular failure predicts a poor survival, liver transplantation would probably be the best therapeutic option.

88 A 45-year-old asymptomatic female is discovered on routine screening to have a titer of antimitochondrial antibodies of >1:160. There are no abnormal findings on clinical examination and her biochemical liver tests are normal.
i. What is the diagnosis?
ii. What other antibodies may be present in her serum?
iii. What is the likely natural history of this patient?

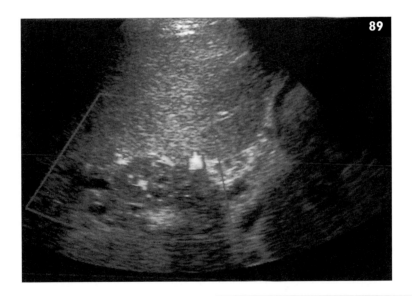

89 A 2-year-old male is noted to have splenomegaly on a routine physical examination. His past history is significant for jaundice and an exchange transfusion via an umbilical catheter during the newborn period. The child has grown well and has no evidence of telangiectasia or palmar erythema. Laboratory investigations are shown.

Total bilirubin 0.6 mg/dL (10.3 µmol/L)
AST 30 U/L
ALT 35 U/L
ALP 153 U/L

i. What does the ultrasound study obtained on this patient (**89**) reveal?
ii. What additional laboratory studies should be performed?
iii. What is the likely diagnosis?

88 i. A titer of antimitochondrial antibodies >1:80 is suggestive of primary biliary cirrhosis. Approximately 90% of patients with primary biliary cirrhosis have detectable titers of antimitochondrial antibodies. The remaining 10% have circulating M2 antibodies which is a more specific and sensitive component of antimitochondrial antibodies. This antibody is directed against the inner component of the mito-chondrial membrane, specifically the pyruvate dehydrogenase complex.

ii. Approximately 20–30% of primary biliary cirrhosis patients have antinuclear antibodies and antibodies against carbonic anhydrase. In addition, primary biliary cirrhosis is associated with other organ specific autoimmune diseases such as scleroderma and thyroid diseases. Antibodies found in these diseases may also be found in the serum.

iii. The majority of patients with positive antimitochondrial antibodies but with normal biochemical liver tests have liver histology characteristic of primary biliary cirrhosis, namely, portal tract granulomata and inflammation. Moreover, most patients progress over 10 years to develop the clinical and biochemical changes of primary biliary cirrhosis.

89 i. Conventional ultrasonography is frequently requested as part of a splenomegaly evaluation. Its noninvasive nature makes it an ideal initial investigation. Doppler ultrasonography allows evaluation of both the patency and direction of portal flow. This study reveals a cavernous transformation of the portal vein with recanalization of the portal vein thrombus and the presence of collateral vessels. In children, cavernous changes can be misinterpreted as portal flow and portal vein obstruction can be missed.

ii. Besides hepatic causes, hematologic and infectious disease problems may result in splenomegaly. It is important to assess the WBC count, hemoglobin or hematocrit, and platelet count as splenomegaly may be associated with the development of hyper-splenism. An enlargement of the spleen is a common clinical sign of portal hyper-tension. When portal pressure increases there is marked congestion and transudation of fluid from the intravascular space into the interstitial tissues of the spleen. The spleen, being highly vascular, enlarges. Other signs of portal hypertension such as ascites, varices, or cutaneous vascular dilations may aid in the diagnosis if there is an intrahepatic cause contributing to the splenomegaly. When congestive splenomegaly exists for a long time, hypersplenism develops. This may result in a decrease in circulating platelets and contribute to bleeding problems.

iii. Cavernous transformation of the portal vein with resultant extrahepatic portal hypertension is the likely diagnosis for this child. Cavernous transformation of the portal vein is defined as the formation of venous channels within or around a previously thrombosed portal vein. The cause of the thrombosis is often obscure although neonatal umbilical vein catheterization, umbilical cord infections, and trauma have been associated with portal vein obstruction. Cardiac and urinary tract anomalies have also been associated with portal vein obstruction. Congenital propensity for thrombus formation caused by protein S, protein C, or antithrombin III deficiencies have also been recognized.

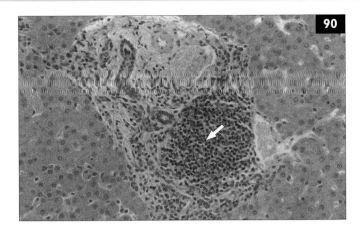

90 A 48-year-old male developed an attack of angina for which he underwent a thorough investigation. Biochemical liver tests revealed an ALT of 184 U/L, AST of 104 U/L, and a positive anti-HCV test result. He denied risk factors for hepatitis. His wife was anti-HCV negative but his brother was found to be anti-HCV positive. Both of his parents died of causes unrelated to hepatitis. The liver was not palpable. His abdominal ultrasound was normal. A liver biopsy was taken. Laboratory investigations are shown.

Bilirubin 0.8 mg/dL (13.68 μmol/L)
Prothrombin time 12.2 seconds
Platelet count 215,000/mm³ (215 × 10⁹/L)
Ferritin 620 ng/mL
Albumin 4.3 g/dL (43 g/L)
Cryoglobulins absent
Tissue antibodies absent
HBsAg absent
HCV-RNA type 1b 1.850 × 10⁶ genomes/mL

i. Describe the liver biopsy findings (90, arrow).
ii. What is the diagnosis?
iii. Comment on the virological data.
iv. What is the natural history of this condition?
v. Should this patient be treated?

91 A 38-year-old Asian male was found on routine blood tests to have elevated aminotransferase values. Viral hepatitis serologies showed reactive HBsAg, anti-HBc, nonreactive HBeAg, anti-HBs, and anti-HCV. The patient denies history of jaundice or hepatitis, transfusions, intravenous drug use, or tattoos.
i. What is the risk for developing hepatocellular carcinoma in this patient?
ii. Should this patient be screened for hepatocellular carcinoma?
iii. Is the patient's family at risk for developing hepatocellular carcinoma?

90 i. The liver biopsy shows enlarged portal tracts with predominantly lymphocytic infiltration. Lymphocytes are arranged in a follicle-like structure. The limiting plate is preserved. Bile ducts are slightly elongated. Liver cells are arranged in regular one-cell-thick plates (H&E).

ii. Community acquired chronic infection with hepatitis C virus leading to chronic hepatitis with minimal to moderate activity.

iii. Viral replication may vary with time, in parallel with recurrent ALT flares. This patient has intermediate levels of viral RNA. The genotype 1b is the most common strain in the Mediterranean area, Europe, and Japan whereas strain 1a predominates in the United States. Patients infected with genotypes 1 and those with higher levels of viremia are less likely to respond to interferon compared to patients infected with other genotypes or with lower viral burden. To date, additional prognostic factors seem to be the patient's age and the presence or absence of cirrhosis.

iv. The natural history of community acquired hepatitis C is still poorly defined. While liver damage during acute infection is usually mild, chronic sequelae may be severe. Chronic hepatitis is a long lasting indolent process which leads to cirrhosis in approximately 20% of cases. There is a subgroup of patients with chronic hepatitis who do not develop cirrhosis or hepatocellular carcinoma. Liver injury or hepatitis C may be accelerated by associated conditions, i.e. coinfection with HIV, allografts, age, and alcohol consumption.

v. Progression to cirrhosis is also demonstrated in patients presenting with mild histological features of chronic hepatitis C. This patient could be offered treatment with pegylated interferon. Ribavirin is relatively contraindicated due to arterio-sclerotic heart disease. If the patient is reluctant to undergo therapy or has an associated condition that makes anti-viral therapy risky such as autoimmune reactions or depression, another option would be to perform a second liver biopsy in 2–3 years time, and to offer treatment only if liver damage has worsened.

91 i. Epidemiologic studies have shown that the risk of developing hepatocellular carcinoma in chronic hepatitis B carriers is 200-fold that of the noninfected population. A prospective study of 22,707 males from Taiwan showed at the 7 year follow-up, 116 cases of hepatocellular carcinoma in the 3,454 males who were HBsAg positive, compared with three cases in the HBsAg negative group.

ii. Yes. The success of a screening program is based on the premise that hepatocellular carcinoma when detected early can be effectively treated with current modalities. By performing serum alphafetoprotein and liver ultrasound examinations every 6 months in chronic hepatitis B virus infected adults over the age of 35, a screening program in China detected 500 cases of hepatocellular carcinoma in 1.3 million people.

iii. Yes. The hepatitis B virus is transmitted by parenteral exposure to bodily fluids of infected patients, as in blood transfusions, sexual intercourse, and close household contacts, particularly in children who more frequently develop chronic infection than adults. Infected women may pass the virus to infants perinatally. Apart from these considerations, there is scanty evidence that hepatocellular carcinoma is hereditary.

92 A 65-year-old chronic alcoholic presents with hematemesis. Physical examination reveals jaundice, spider angiomata, tense ascites, melena, and asterixis.

Laboratory investigations are shown. Upper endoscopy reveals actively bleeding, grade IV esophageal varices which are successfully sclerosed.

Hemoglobin 8.2 g/dL (82 g/L)
Prothrombin time 16.4 seconds
AST 80 U/L
ALT 20 U/L
Albumin 2.4 g/dL (24 g/L)
Total bilirubin 4.2 mg/dL (71.8 μmol/L)
ALP 112 U/L
GGTP 200 U/L

i. Assuming that the variceal bleeding can be adequately controlled, what is a major determinant of this patient's prognosis?
ii. What effective therapy is available for this patient?
iii. What is the role of liver transplantation for this patient?

93 A patient undergoes liver transplantation for chronic alcoholic cirrhosis and has an hepatic artery thrombosis 3 days later. Revascularization is successfully undertaken. She does well thereafter and is discharged. At a follow-up visit 3 months later, she is jaundiced and the results of laboratory investigations are shown. Duplex ultrasound reveals a patent hepatic artery and portal vein. An ERCP film is obtained (93). The most likely diagnosis is:
A Biliary leak.
B Hepatitis.
C Rejection.
D Ischemic stricture.

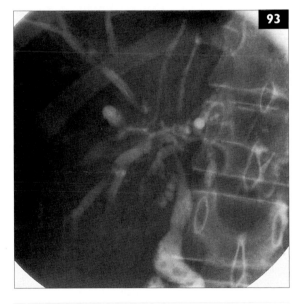

Bilirubin 5.2 mg/dL (88.92 μmol/L)
Prothrombin time 11.5 seconds
AST 45 U/L

92 i. The mere presence of cirrhosis does not always indicate a poor prognosis, and frequently its presence is not suspected. Continuing alcohol abuse and the coexistence of alcoholic hepatitis (which requires alcohol use) are important prognostic factors. Similar to the discriminant function formula devised for alcoholic hepatitis, a combined clinical and laboratory index has been developed for patients with cirrhosis which includes the presence or absence of various clinical abnormalities (hepatic encephalopathy, collateral circulation, edema, ascites, spider nevi, weakness, and anorexia) and the degree of abnormality of various laboratory tests (prothrombin time, hematocrit, albumin level, bilirubin, and ALP concentrations) that identifies patients at a high risk of death within 1 year.

ii. Abstinence is critical in patients with alcoholic cirrhosis as it prolongs survival, even in patients with symptoms of portal hypertension and hepatic insufficiency. Nutritional therapy is also important. Intensive dietary supplementation is associated with increased serum albumin levels, improved Child's scores, a lower risk of death in hospitalized patients, and a decreased rate of hospitalization for severe infections in outpatients.

iii. In 1983 a National Institute of Health Consensus Development Panel concluded that orthotopic liver transplantation is an appropriate option for patients with alcoholic cirrhosis in whom liver failure progresses and life threatening complications develop despite abstinence from alcohol. The means to predict which patients are likely to remain sober are controversial. Many transplant centers require that patients demonstrate a clear understanding of his/her alcoholism and undergo a rehabilitation program with a period of abstinence.

93 D. Ischemic stricture. Twenty-five per cent of the blood supply to the liver comes from the hepatic artery origin and 75% from the portal vein. The portal blood carries less well oxygenated blood, providing about 50% of the oxygen supply. However, the entire blood supply to the biliary tree derives from the hepatic artery, the radicles of which run within a thin fibrous sheath that represents a continuation of Glisson's capsule. This peribiliary plexus of arterioles nourishes the biliary ductal system. Hepatic artery thrombosis occurs in 4–15% of cases of liver transplantation and usually results in ischemic necrosis of the allograft. If the thrombosis is promptly diagnosed and revascularization is accomplished, the graft may be salvaged. Late sequelae of such procedures can include ischemic-type biliary strictures, or areas of liver necrosis and bile collections within the liver parenchyma. In the ERCP shown, the arrows point to diffuse intrahepatic stricturing of the biliary tree most consistent with ischemic injury. Prolonged pretransplant cold ischemic time can produce a similar picture. Duplex ultrasound revealing a patent artery suggests that this arose from a prior episode in the perioperative period. The therapeutic options in cases such as this are limited. If stricture formation is focal, then a combination of endoscopic or radiologic dilation sometimes relieves obstruction. Balloon dilation or placement of an expandable stent are therapeutic options. If the stricture is extrahepatic, then biliary reconstruction to a jejunal limb may accomplish drainage. If stricturing is diffuse throughout the biliary tree, retransplantation will ultimately be required, either to control recurrent cholangitis or when biliary obstruction leads to the eventual development of secondary biliary cirrhosis.

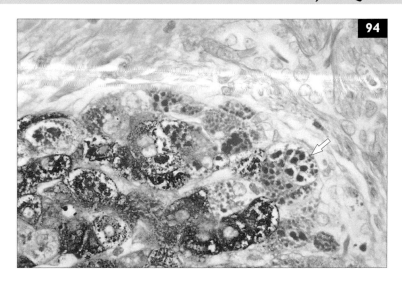

94 A patient with a low alpha-1-globulin level on serum protein electrophoresis is suspected of having alpha-1-antitrypsin deficiency. A liver biopsy is performed to confirm the diagnosis and assess the degree of liver injury.
i. What is revealed by the liver biopsy (**94**, arrow)?
ii. What therapy is available?
iii. What is the prognosis for this patient?

95 A 19-year-old female was seen because she developed fatigue, jaundice, hepatomegaly, and ALT activity 15 times the upper limit of normal. She tested negative for hepatitis A, B, and C and denied intravenous drug exposure or alcohol use. Aminotransferase activities remained 10 times the upper limit of normal for 6 months and the patient underwent a liver biopsy which showed hepatitis. Two years later, the patient developed fatigue, and ALT 40 times the upper limit of normal. Abdominal ultrasound examination shows a normal sized liver with a slight increase of echopatterns and a normal sized spleen. Laboratory investigations are shown.

Bilirubin 1.8 mg/dL (30.8 μmol/L)
Prothrombin time 12.4 seconds
ALP 414 U/L
Platelet count 287,000/mm³ (287 × 10⁹/L)
Ceruloplasmin 29 mg/dL (290 mg/L)
Smooth muscle antibodies 1: 80
Anti-HCV absent
HBsAg absent
Gammaglobulin 4.1 g/dL (41 g/L)
Antimitochondrial antibody absent
Antinuclear antibodies 1:160 homogeneous
IgM anti-HAV absent
Liver–kidney microsomal antibodies absent

i. What is the diagnosis?
ii. Comment on the classification and disease specificity of tissue antibodies.

94 i. This biopsy depicts the distinctive PAS-positive diastase-resistant globules in the endoplasmic reticulum of hepatocytes in alpha-1-antitrypsin deficiency, a common genetic disorder affecting about 1 in 1,800 live births in North America and Northern Europe. It is an autosomal recessive disorder that causes an 85% reduction in circulating levels of alpha-1-antitrypsin in serum, premature emphysema, chronic liver disease progressing to cirrhosis and portal hypertension, and even hepatocellular carcinoma. Liver involvement is usually recognized in the first 2 months of life as persistent jaundice. Serum aminotransferase activities are elevated and hepatomegaly may be appreciated.

ii. No specific therapy is available for the liver disease associated with alpha-1-antitrypsin deficiency. It is helpful to identify infants at risk and provide genetic counselling to family members. Genetically engineered alpha-1-antitrypsin has been administered intravenously to adults with emphysema secondary to alpha-1-antitrypsin deficiency with improvement in pulmonary function. As the hepatic injury in alpha-1-antitrypsin deficiency is caused by the presence of abnormal alpha-1-antitrypsin globules in hepatocytes, intravenous infusion of alpha-1-antitrypsin does not correct the hepatic defect. Patients heterozygous or homozygous for alpha-1-antitrypsin deficiency should be cautioned about smoking and alcohol consumption as several reports have linked these behaviors with a more rapid disease course.

iii. The prognosis of alpha-1-antitrypsin deficiency is extremely variable. The hepatocellular cholestasis, jaundice, and hepatomegaly observed in the newborn period often dissipates over a few months after birth. Occasionally, fulminant hepatic failure and death occur unless the child undergoes liver transplantation. More commonly, biliary cirrhosis and portal hypertension develop within 5–15 years. Liver transplantation has been successfully used in children with cirrhosis and portal hypertension caused by alpha-1-antitrypsin deficiency. The recipient assumes the alpha-1-antitrypsin phenotype of the donor liver. Not all patients with homozygous alpha-1-antitrypsin deficiency develop liver or lung disease.

95 i. The 6 months duration of symptoms, three to 10-fold elevations in aminotransferase activities, gammaglobulin concentrations twice normal, high titer (>1:40) tissue antibodies, and exclusion of all other etiological factors indicate autoimmune hepatitis, type I with severe chronic active hepatitis.

ii. Autoimmune hepatitis type I is characterized by the presence of antinuclear antibodies, often accompanied by smooth muscle antibodies. Under immunofluorescence examination, antinuclear antibodies show a homogenous nuclear reactivity in contrast to the speckled pattern of virus- or drug-induced antinuclear antibodies reactivities. Autoimmune hepatitis type II is characterized by liver-kidney microsomal antibodies type I (LKM_1) that are directed against a short linear sequence of P450 2D6, a drug metabolizing enzyme system. Autoimmune hepatitis type III is characterized by antibodies against soluble liver antigens. These antibodies are directed against cytokeratins 8 and 18. The presence of antinuclear antibodies and smooth muscle antibodies, defining autoimmune hepatitis I, is mutually exclusive of the occurrence of anti-LKM_1 which defines autoimmune hepatitis II.

96 A 67-year-old Caucasian male presented with hematemesis. Upper endoscopy showed blood clots in the stomach and esophageal varices which were not actively bleeding. He underwent banding of the varices. Abdominal ultrasound examination showed a small heterogeneous liver consistent with cirrhosis, and mild splenomegaly. Blood tests were positive for antibodies to hepatitis C virus.
i. What is the risk for developing hepatocellular carcinoma in this patient?
ii. Should this patient be screened for hepatocellular carcinoma?
iii. Is there treatment to prevent the development of hepatocellular carcinoma in this patient?
iv. Is the patient's family at risk for developing hepatocellular carcinoma?

97 A 4-month-old female is seen by her pediatrician because of parental concerns for an abdominal mass. Physical examination reveals hepatomegaly and congestive heart failure. A bruit is heard over the liver. A small strawberry hemangioma is noted on her back. Laboratory investigations are shown.
i. Comment on the ultrasound study (97a).
ii. What does the biopsy reveal (97b)?

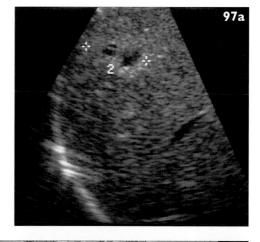

Hemoglobin 9 g/dL (90 g/L)
Platelet count 50,000/mm³
(50 × 10⁹/L)
AST 130 U/L

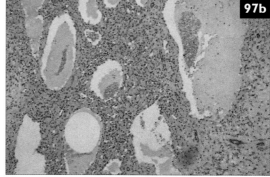

96 i. Case control studies have shown a close epidemiologic association of hepatitis C infection and hepatocellular carcinoma. The prevalence of anti-HCV positivity in patients with hepatocellular carcinoma is substantially higher than in the control population. Up to 60–70% of Japanese hepatocellular carcinoma patients are positive for antibodies to hepatitis C virus. Studies of transfusion-related hepatitis C infection have documented the progression from acute to chronic hepatitis to cirrhosis and to hepatocellular carcinoma after 7–23 years. Unlike hepatitis B virus related hepatocellular carcinoma, where up to 27% of cases occur in noncirrhotic livers, nearly all cases of hepatitis C virus related hepatocellular carcinoma are associated with cirrhosis.

ii. No reports of screening programs for hepatocellular carcinoma in hepatitis C virus infected patients have been published. Unlike hepatitis B virus, hepatitis C virus related hepatocellular carcinomas are more frequently multifocal and occur nearly exclusively in patients with cirrhosis. Local regional treatment modalities such as surgical resection or alcohol injection for early hepatocellular carcinoma are, therefore, expected to be less effective, which may affect the success of screening programs in prolonging survival for hepatitis C virus infected patients.

iii. No. Interferon-alpha/ribavirin has been effective in improving serum aminotransferase values, reducing hepatic necroinflammation, and eradicating detectable serum hepatitis C virus-RNA in patients with chronic hepatitis C virus infection. The efficacy of interferon-based therapy in preventing hepatocellular carcinoma remains under investigation. There are reports of a lower incidence of the development of hepatocellular carcinoma in patients treated with interferon, even in patients without viral elimination. Confirmation of this observation is needed.

iv. No. No familial clustering or genetic predisposition to hepatocellular carcinoma has been indentified in patients chronically infected with hepatitis C virus. The primary risk factors in hepatitis C virus transmission is via parenteral exposure to infected blood and blood products, as occurs with sharing needles and blood transfusions.

97 i. This ultrasound study reveals an hepatic abnormality consistent with a vascular lesion. Diagnostic imaging is helpful in the evaluation of abdominal masses. Ultrasound examination may reveal single or multiple hyperechoic, complex, or hypoechoic lesions. A CT scan may show the hepatic origin of the lesion, whether it is single or multifocal, and whether it extends outside the liver. Selective angiography may demonstrate diffuse angiomatous lesions with rapid filling of the hepatic vein. Chest radiography may demonstrate cardiomegaly with or without pulmonary vascular prominence.

ii. This biopsy specimen is composed of vascular channels lined by a singular continuous layer of plump endothelial cells in a supporting fibrous stroma. The tumors are single in about half of the cases and multiple in the rest. Single lesions may be small or large and equally distributed between the right and left hepatic lobes. If near the liver surface the lesions may show central umbilication. On cut section they are well demarcated, reddish-brown to light tan, and soft and spongy. In large lesions, central areas of infarction, hemorrhage, fibrosis, and yellowish gritty specks of calcification may be present.

98 With regard to the case in 97:
i. What is the likely diagnosis?
ii. What treatment do you advise?

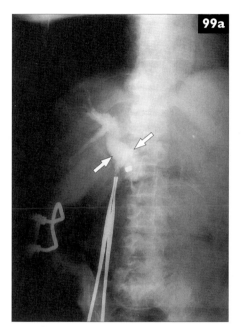

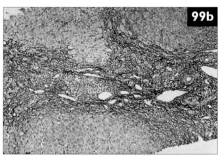

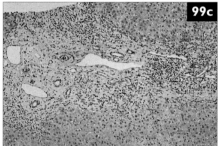

99 A patient with a history of chronic alcohol abuse underwent an exploratory laparotomy to evaluate and drain an obstructed biliary tree. An intraoperative cholangiogram was obtained.
i. Comment on the radiograph of the bile duct ((99a, arrows).
ii. What do the liver biopsies show (99b, c)?
iii. What is the pathophysiology of this complication of alcohol abuse?
iv. What differential diagnosis should be considered in evaluating this biliary abnormality?
v. How should this patient be managed?

98 i. The likely diagnosis is an infantile hemangioendothelioma. Infantile hemangioendothelioma is the most common benign tumor of the liver in children. It is the most common liver tumor seen in children <1 year old. It clinically often presents as an abdominal mass with jaundice, respiratory symptoms, congestive heart failure, and skin hemangiomas. Lesions may be single or multiple. There is a slight female preponderance. Jaundice, heart failure, and thrombocytopenia may suggest a poor prognosis. The Kasabach–Merritt syndrome refers to thrombocytopenia and hypofibrinogenemia with consumptive coagulopathy. The coagulopathy is attributed to the trapping and destruction of platelets within the vascular tumor with progression to disseminated intravascular coagulation, and activation of clotting and fibrinolytic pathways. Hemangiomas may be present on the skin or in other visceral organs.
ii. Treatment is dependent upon the symptomatology and whether the lesion is single or multifocal. Surgical excision is advocated for single lesions or lesions amenable to lobectomy. Patients with congestive heart failure must be treated with cardiac medication such as digoxin and diuretics. Steroid administration may be helpful in speeding up the regression of the tumor and improving the platelet count and may be required for many months of therapy. Radiation therapy has been used in the past but is in disfavor because of the potential for long term side effects. Low dose cytoxan and interferon therapy may be useful in selected cases. Hepatic artery ligation and transarterial embolization have also been used but may result in significant morbidity and mortality if there is tremendous tumor necrosis.

99 i. Dilation of the common bile duct is confirmed.
ii. The liver biopsies reveal changes of biliary obstruction with proliferation of bile ductules and portal fibrosis (Trichrome stain **99b, c**).
iii. Chronic partial obstruction of the common bile duct can complicate chronic calcific pancreatitis and lead to progressive biliary fibrosis and cirrhosis.
iv. A carcinoma in the head of the pancreas in chronic pancreatitis mimicking a benign stricture is also a possibility.
v. In one large study, chronic common bile duct stenosis complicated 8% of patients with alcoholic pancreatitis who were screened biochemically for an ALP elevation greater than twofold for at least 1 month. Most of the patients with this complication were anicteric and asymptomatic except for their symptoms of pancreatitis. Varying degrees of biliary obstructive histopathology, as illustrated by this patient's liver biopsy, were present in 79% of the cases. Less frequently, histologic cholangitis was also present. The degree of bilirubin and ALP elevation did not correlate with stricture length or the severity of bile duct obstruction. Approximately one third of the cases had secondary biliary cirrhosis, and progression was documented in several patients with sequential biopsies. As a result, it is recommended that biliary decompression be considered in patients with persistent common bile duct stenosis from alcoholic pancreatitis, especially if there are recurrent attacks of septic cholangitis or if biliary cirrhosis is present.

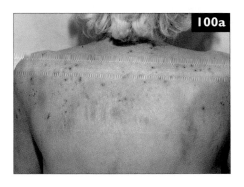
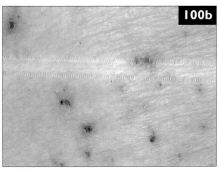

100 A 92-year-old female was admitted via the emergency room with a 3 day history of fever, back pain, and icteric sclerae. She denied recent travel and contact with anyone with known illnesses. She had a cholecystectomy 9 years ago for what appeared to be cholecystitis associated with jaundice. She had a T-tube in the common bile duct for several days after surgery. She reported having suffered from pruritus for 2 years which had not been relieved by the antipruritic medications that had been prescribed. Physical examination was significant for icteric sclerae, surgical abdominal scars, and right costophrenic angle tenderness to palpation. Her skin revealed several pustular lesions and areas of excoriations (100a, b). CT scans of the abdomen revealed the absence of a gallbladder and no dilated intrahepatic ducts. There was a 2 cm (0.8 in) lesion in the capsular region of the right kidney consistent with an abscess which was aspirated. The material removed grew *Staphylococcus aureus*. Blood cultures taken on admission grew the same organism. On antibiotic treatment the patient defervesced and her bilirubin decreased to normal. However, her liver profile remained cholestatic. Her pruritus persisted. Laboratory investigations are shown.

i. How can transient jaundice be explained in this patient?
ii. In view of her persistent cholestasis, what diagnostic test is in order?
iii. Why is this patient pruritic?
iv. What treatment would you recommend?

	Day 1	Day 6	Day 20*	Day 30**
ALP (U/L)	674	759	821	520
Total bilirubin (mg/dL [μmol/L])	4.9 (83.8)	9.1 (155.6)	5.1 (87.2)	1.0 (17.1)
Direct bilirubin (mg/dL [μmol/L])	4.2 (71.8)	6.9 (118.0)	3.5 (59.9)	0.5 (8.6)
AST (U/L)	42	38	76	34
ALT (U/L)	37	46	55	32
Cholesterol (mg/dL [mmol/L])	483 (12.5)	695 (18)	537 (13.9)	430 (11.1)

* 10 days after completion of antibiotic therapy
** 20 days after completion of antibiotic therapy

100 i. Transient jaundice may be explained by the syndrome of cholestasis of sepsis.
ii. Cholangiography is indicated, either magnetic resonance choliangiography (MRCP) or ERCP.
iii. Cholestasis can cause pruritus. The history of cholecystectomy and T-tube placement in the postoperative period suggests a complicated procedure. Complicated cholecystectomies may result in biliary tract strictures (e.g. common bile duct) with subsequent cholestasis and secondary biliary cirrhosis. Her history of chronic pruritus is consistent with a cholestatic syndrome and it is substantiated by her skin findings which include multiple excoriations and prurigo nodularis. Presumably the source of her *Staphyloccocus aureus* sepsis was infected skin lesions. The hyperbilirubinemia during the sepsis which subsided after adequate treatment and resolution of the infection can be explained by the syndrome of cholestasis of sepsis. The incidence of cholestasis associated with sepsis of nonhepatobiliary origin has been reported in the literature to be as high as 50%. It tends to appear within a few days of onset of bacteremia. Hepatomegaly may be seen in 50% of patients. Serum bilirubin, primarily conjugated, peaks between 5–10 mg/dL (85.5–171.0 µmol/L) and serum ALP may be elevated in 50% of the cases. Serum aminotransferase activities may be elevated or normal. Liver biopsy, which is not necessary to make the diagnosis, reveals intrahepatic cholestasis with little or no hepatocellular necrosis. Cholestasis of sepsis is more commonly seen in sepsis caused by Gram-negative organisms although it can be seen in cases of sepsis caused by Gram-positive organisms as was the case in this patient. *In vivo* and *in vitro* animal studies on the cholestasis of sepsis reveal an inhibitory effect of transport mechanisms by lipopolysaccharide including: the inhibition of the activity of Na^+ K^+ adenosine triphosphatase (ATPase) which is involved in the bile-acid independent fraction of bile secretion, inhibition of canalicular transport of organic anions, and inhibition of hepatocellular sodium-dependent bile salt uptake by a decrease in the expression of Ntcp, a sodium-dependent bile acid (taurocholate) cotransporter. In addition, intravenous infusions of lipotechoic acid, a component of the cellular wall of Gram-positive organisms (e.g. *Staphylococci*) is associated with retention of bromosulphthalein in rabbits.
iv. The treatment of cholestasis of sepsis is to remove the underlying infection. In this patient, however, the liver profile remained cholestatic, in spite of resolution of sepsis and normalization of bilirubin. In view of the history of cholecystectomy a cholangiogram is indicated to rule out the presence of postsurgical biliary stricture. Intraoperative bile duct injury may not be immediately recognized and it may present clinically several years after the surgery with cholestasis and, or, episodes of cholangitis. The treatment of this complication is surgical repair by an experienced surgeon or endoscopic balloon dilation and possible stent placement.

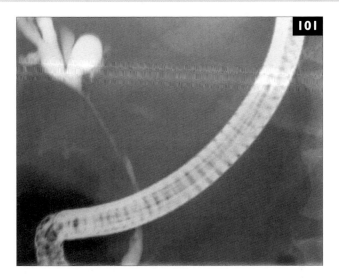

101 An 84-year-old female presents with painless obstructive jaundice. A percutaneous transabdominal ultrasound shows dilation of the intrahepatic ducts but the common bile duct is not visualized.
i. What does the ERCP (101) show?
ii. What is the differential diagnosis?
iii. What treatment is indicated?

102 A full term, 8.8 lb (4 kg) birthweight, newborn male is delivered to a 34-year-old female. The pregnancy was notable for elevated maternal aminotransferase values during the first prenatal visit at 12 weeks gestation. During the 15th week, serum aminotransferase values peaked with ALT 450 U/L and AST 250 U/L. This improved to an ALT of 55 U/L and AST of 50 U/L during the third trimester. The mother was found to be HBsAg positive during her routine prenatal screen. She did not recall any previous symptoms of hepatitis, denied intravenous drug use, blood transfusions, or sexual or intimate exposure. There is no family history of hepatitis. Subsequent laboratory studies revealed IgG anti-HBc. Serologies for other hepatitis viruses and HIV were all nonreactive.
i. When should prenatal screening for hepatitis B occur?
ii. What therapy should be given to this newborn child whose mother is hepatitis B positive?
iii. Do children whose mothers are not infected with hepatitis B need hepatitis B immunization?
iv. Can this mother safely breast feed her child if she desires?

101 i. A long common bile stricture also involving the hepatic duct to the level of the bifurcation of the biliary tree.

ii. The most likely diagnosis in this clinical context is cholangiocarcinoma. Extensive infiltration by pancreatic cancer is possible but less likely. Benign disease such as primary sclerosing cholangitis is possible but the dilation of the biliary tree makes this unlikely. The diagnosis is that of cholangiocarcinoma. There are associations with chronic infection by biliary parasites such as clinorchis, with primary sclerosing cholangitis, previous exposure to thorotrast, and choledochal cyst. There is a poor association with gallstones although these are strongly associated with the development of gallbladder cancer. The adenocarcinoma may be diffuse or nodular and sclerosing.

iii. In this elderly patient operative treatment is not indicated and the results of surgical resection are poor. Stenting either by the endoscopic or percutaneous route is indicated. There is a little evidence that intracavity irradiation using iridium wires may halt progression of the disease.

102 i. Hepatitis B screening early during pregnancy allows identification of infected mothers and allows proper treatment of the newborn.

ii. To provide maximum protection, an infant born to an HBsAg positive mother should receive the first dose of hepatitis B vaccine and hepatitis B immune globulin within 12 hours of birth. Without protection, up to 90% of infants born to mothers who are positive for HBsAg and show evidence of viral replication (HBeAg positive or hepatitis B virus-DNA positive) will contract acute hepatitis B. Of these infants, 80–90% will remain chronically infected.

iii. The Centers for Disease Control and Prevention and the American Academy of Pediatrics have recommended universal immunization of all children in the United States including newborn infants, children, and adolescents whose mothers are not infected with hepatitis B in an attempt to eradicate hepatitis B. The risk of chronic hepatitis B and liver disease is greatest when the infection occurs perinatally or during early childhood. Children whose mothers are not infected with hepatitis B virus should receive the hepatitis B vaccine series alone with the first dose preferably given in the newborn nursery before discharge home. If a mother is unscreened or originally negative for hepatitis B and subsequently found to be positive for HBsAg, the infant should receive hepatitis B immune globulin within the first 7 days of birth. If not administered in this time frame, then the second dose of hepatitis B vaccine should be given at 1 month of age because of the high risk for chronic infection. The last dose of the initial vaccine series should be given at 6 months of age.

iv. Once this child has received the first dose of hepatitis B vaccine and hepatitis B immune globulin, it is safe for this mother to proceed with breast feeding if she desires to do so. Breast milk contains many beneficial immunologic and growth factors unavailable in infant formula.

103 A 24-year-old primigravid, Caucasian female at 36 weeks presents with a 10 day history of nausea, vomiting, malaise, and worsening right upper quadrant abdominal pain. She has no itch and has taken no medications. Examination reveals normal blood pressure, modest jaundice, a gravid abdomen with mild right upper quadrant tenderness, no

Bilirubin 4.1 mg/dL (70.1 µmol/L)
ALT 300 U/L
Albumin 2.9 g/dL (29 g/L)
WBC count 15,000/mm³ (15 x 10⁹/l)
Hemoglobin normal
Platelet count normal
Fibrinogen decreased

palpable liver or spleen, and no ankle edema. Laboratory investigations are shown. An upper abdominal percutaneous ultrasound shows a small liver, no gallstones or common bile duct dilation, and a normal spleen.
i. What other history is particularly relevant here?
ii. What is the diagnosis and what other tests may help?
iii. Is a liver biopsy indicated and what histology is expected?
iv. What is the best course of treatment?
v. Does she risk recurrence in subsequent pregnancies?

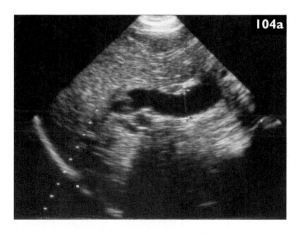

104 A 54-year-old male with a long history of alcoholism complicated by chronic, calcific pancreatitis presents with abnormal liver tests. Laboratory investigations are shown. A percutaneous abdominal ultrasound was obtained (**104a**).

Comment on the ultrasound findings and suggest further evaluation.

Hemoglobin 14.2 g/dL (142 g/L)
MCV 102.4 fL (mm³)
Prothrombin time 14.2
AST 80 U/L
ALT 28 U/L
Albumin 3.8 g/dL (38 g/L)
Total bilirubin 1.8 mg/dL (30.8 µmol/L)
ALP 412 U/L
GGTP 820 U/L
Amylase 80 U/L

103 i. A detailed travel history is important because viral hepatitis can mimic this presentation.

ii. The low fibrinogen with normal hemoglobin and platelets, small liver with normal spleen and vessels, and increased aminotransferase activities imply hepatocyte injury. The most likely diagnosis is acute fatty liver of pregnancy, suggested by jaundice, a small liver, and characteristic physical examination and blood tests. There are no features of pre-eclampsia in 50% of acute fatty liver of pregnancy cases. The risk of acute fatty liver of pregnancy complicating pregnancy increases with multiple gestation (e.g. twins) or first pregnancy. Up to 80% of patients can present with abdominal pain and vomiting but the presentation may be nonspecific malaise and anorexia. The etiology is related to a metabolic disturbance of the mitochondrial urea cycle enzymes in the liver. The mode of initiation in the third trimester is unknown. Ammonia levels may be elevated as hepatocytes fail but is not especially specific or sensitive for liver disease. Glucose levels are often low in acute fatty liver of pregnancy but again this is not specific. High serum urate levels are usual and not commonly found in other forms of liver failure.

iii. Liver biopsy is sometimes indicated to confirm the diagnosis e.g. to assist management in atypical presentations when the pregnancy is <36 weeks and there is concern about fetal survival. Typical liver histology shows microvesicular steatosis in centrizonal hepatocytes with or without patchy hepatocellular necrosis. Other causes of microvesicular fat include tetracycline, sodium valproate toxicity, and Reye's syndrome. The histology can be more subtle and mimic viral hepatitis or obstructive cholangitis. Usually the histology returns to normal with no long term sequelae after delivery.

iv. The fetus should be delivered without delay because acute fatty liver of pregnancy is life threatening for both mother and baby, as liver dysfunction and disseminated intravascular coagulation can progress rapidly. Great care must be taken postpartum as liver and renal failure may progress up to 1–2 weeks following delivery. Some patients with advanced liver failure have successfully undergone orthotopic liver transplantation for this condition.

v. Acute fatty liver of pregnancy is not any more likely in subsequent pregnancies.

104 The abdominal ultrasound reveals a dilated common bile duct. An abdominal CT scan is indicated to further evaluate the cause of biliary obstruction. The CT scan demonstrates changes consistent with chronic pancreatitis with calcifications and pancreatic duct dilation(**104b**, arrow).

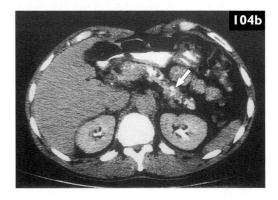

105 On a routine check-up, a lean 25-year-old male was found to have abnormal biochemical liver test results. He feels well and does not have any symptoms of liver disease. He is not taking any medication, has no history of blood transfusions, and has never taken intravenous drugs. Laboratory investigations are shown.

Hemoglobin 13 g/dL (130 g/L)
WBC count 8,000/mm³ (8 × 10⁹/L)
Platelet count 305,000/mm³ (305 × 10⁹/L)
ESR 10 mm/hour
AST 72 U/L
ALT 88 U/L
ALP 280 U/L
Bilirubin 1.34 mg/dL (23 μmol/L)
Albumin 4 g/dL (40 g/L)
Prothrombin time normal
Serology for hepatitis A, B, and C negative

i. What further serological tests do you suggest?
ii. What further investigations do you suggest?

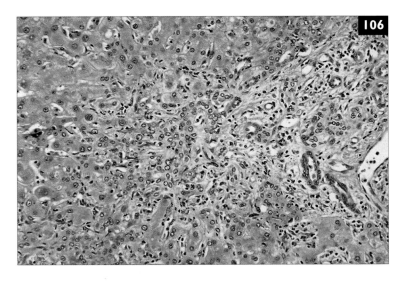

106 A liver biopsy was performed in a 2-month-old patient being evaluated for the new onset of jaundice while on TPN. An extensive evaluation including a review of the medical history for drugs or transfusion exposures was negative. Abdominal ultrasound examination was normal. Serum protein electrophoresis and a metabolic screen were normal.
i. Comment on the histologic findings (**106**).
ii. What treatment is recommended for TPN associated cholestasis?

105 i. This young, asymptomatic male shows the biochemical signs of cholestasis. In order to exclude primary biliary cirrhosis and chronic autoimmune hepatitis, tests aiming at detecting mitochondrial autoantibodies, smooth muscle antibodies, and antinuclear antibodies should be carried out. Furthermore, an electrophoresis should be undertaken for immunoglobulin levels. Ceruloplasmin levels and alpha-1-antitrypsin phenotype should be determined. This patient had no mitochondrial or smooth muscle antibodies but an antinuclear antibody test was positive in a titer of 1 in 80. The levels of immunoglobulins, alpha-1-antitrypsin phenotype, and ceruloplasmin were normal. Thus, there is no evidence

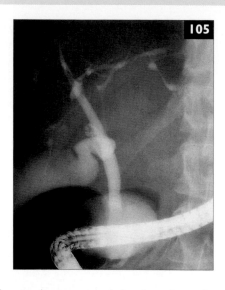

to suggest primary biliary cirrhosis, Wilson's disease, or alpha-1-antitrypsin deficiency. Although a slight increase in antinuclear antibodies was found, the normal IgG level makes chronic autoimmune hepatitis unlikely.

ii. An ultrasound investigation and a liver biopsy should be performed. The liver biopsy for this patient showed periportal inflammation and concentric fibrosis around the bile ducts ('onion lesions'). This histological finding is typical of primary sclerosing cholangitis, but an ERCP has to be undertaken to make a definitive diagnosis. It was found that this man had multifocal strictures and irregularities diffusely distributed in the intrahepatic bile ducts (**105**). These findings are compatible with a diagnosis of primary sclerosing cholangitis. As primary sclerosing cholangitis is closely associated with inflammatory bowel disease, all patients with primary sclerosing cholangitis must undergo colonoscopic investigation with biopsies in the search of evidence for ulcerative colitis or Crohn's disease. Colonoscopy revealed total ulcerative colitis despite an absence of symptoms.

106 i. The biopsy specimen shows intralobular cholestasis with an inflammatory portal tract lesion. There is bile stasis, as evidenced by a bile plug, and mild to moderate bile duct proliferation. In addition there is evidence of periportal fibrosis.

ii. Prevention is the key to treatment for TPN associated liver disease. Appropriate calorie intake with adequate mixtures of carbohydrates, protein, and fat are essential. Enteral feedings even if only in minimal amounts should be instituted as soon as possible. Weekly monitoring laboratory studies should be obtained. If cholestasis is evident enteral feeding should be aggressively attempted. If bacterial overgrowth is suspected, appropriate antibiotic therapy should be instituted. Cholecystokinin and ursodeoxycholic acid have been used in some patients to stimulate bile flow with mixed results.

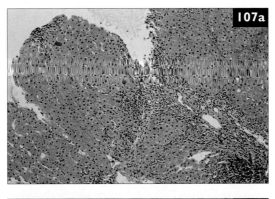

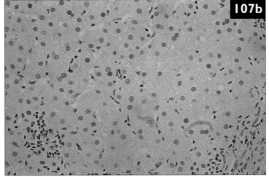

107 A 32-year-old female presents with fatigue and a 10 year history of elevated serum aminotransferase activities. HBsAg is detectable in her serum. She admits to intravenous drug use at the age of 18, but denies alcohol intake. Examination reveals moderate hepatosplenomegaly and spider angiomata. Laboratory investigations are shown. Abdominal ultrasound shows moderate hepatosplenomegaly with increased echopattern of the liver.

i. Describe the liver histology (107a).
ii. The liver biopsy was reacted with anti-HD. Comment on the immunohistologic staining pattern of the liver (107b).
iii. What is the diagnosis?
iv. What is the epidemiology and the natural history of this disease?
v. What further investigations are appropriate?
vi. What is the ideal therapy and follow-up of this patient?
vii. Can this disease be prevented?

Bilirubin 0.5 mg/dL (8.6 µmol/L)
ALT 132 U/L
AST 86 U/L
Albumin 4.3 g/dL (43 g/L)
Platelet count 135,000/mm³ (135 × 10⁹/L)
HBsAg present
Anti-HBe present
HBeAg absent
Hepatitis B virus-DNA absent
IgG anti-HD 1:4,000
IgM anti-HD present

107 i. The liver biopsy shows architectural distortion with portal–central bridging. Portal tracts are accentuated by increased numbers of chronic inflammatory cells. There is severe piecemeal periportal necrosis.

ii. Nuclei of several liver cells stained brown with antibody to hepatitis D virus antigen conjugated with horseradish peroxidase. This technique allows for identification of the antigen in the infected liver cells and is a reliable signal of ongoing hepatitis D virus replication.

iii. Chronic infection with hepatitis D virus and hepatitis B leading to chronic hepatitis and cirrhosis. The diagnosis of hepatitis D virus infection relies on detection of serum antibody to the hepatitis D virus antigen (IgG and IgM). Infection can be directly diagnosed by tests for hepatitis D virus-RNA in serum and hepatitis D virus antigen in the liver.

iv. Hepatitis D virus is a defective RNA viral agent which requires helper functions of hepatitis B virus for essential parts of its life cycle. The pathogenic mechanisms of hepatitis D virus are unknown but may involve direct cytopathic events associated with virus replication and expression. Unlike hepatitis B virus, hepatitis D virus infects only the liver cells, it causes both acute and chronic hepatitis. Hepatitis B virus contributes its envelope to form the exterior structure of hepatitis D virus, thereby providing extracellular stability and a means of liver cell entry. Transmission can occur either by coinfection of a hepatitis B virus susceptible person or by superinfection of a hepatitis B virus carrier. Infection has been transmitted by the parenteral route (transfusions and intravenous drug abuse), sexual exposure, or family contact. Neonatal transmission of hepatitis D virus is exceptional. Hepatitis D virus often results in severe acute or fulminant hepatitis and leads to chronic liver disease. Chronic infection, after hepatitis D virus coinfection, occurs in <10% of patients while superinfection leads to cirrhosis in 20% of the patients within 4 years.

v. Upper gastrointestinal endoscopy to look for esophageal varices.

vi. The only therapeutic agent found to be active against hepatitis D virus is interferon-alpha. High doses of interferon (6 MU or more) for 6–12 months provided some transient benefits to 30–50% of the patients. Sustained responses were found to be rare. Liver transplantation is the ideal treatment for patients with decompensated cirrhosis as the risk of reinfection is lower than for hepatitis B virus alone or hepatitis C virus. Prophylaxis with hyperimmune HBIg may improve the outlook after transplantation. The 5 year survival rate was 88% in one series of 76 patients.

vii. Hepatitis D virus infection can be avoided by preventing hepatitis B virus infection with the hepatitis B vaccine.

108 A 23-year-old female medical student developed dark urine, fever, and abdominal discomfort 3 weeks after returning from an elective in India. She has not taken any recent medication. Laboratory investigations are shown.
i. What is the most likely diagnosis?
ii. What are the possible clinical outcomes?

Bilirubin 5.85 mg/dL (100 μmol/L)	
Albumin 4.4 g/dL (44 g/L)	
ALT 1,120 U/L	
ALP 120 U/L	
Prothrombin time 14 seconds	

109 A 28-year-old female was admitted to the hospital with right upper quadrant pain with radiation to the left upper quadrant and back. The pain was associated with nausea and vomiting. The patient had no past history of liver disease or use of alcohol, but had taken oral contraceptives for 8 years. Laboratory investigations are shown. The patient was found dead in bed 4 hours after hospital admission.
i. Describe the gross autopsy findings (**109a**).
ii. Describe the histologic findings (**109b**).
iii. What would a CT scan of the liver have shown if performed?
iv. With what lesion is this condition often confused and how is the natural history different?

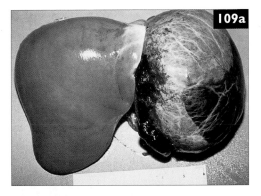

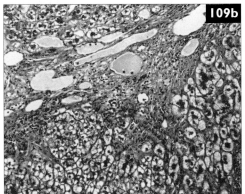

Hematocrit 34%
WBC count 10,200/mm³ (10.2 × 10⁹/L)
Platelet count 157,000/mm³ (157 × 10⁹/L)
AST 766 U/L
LDH 832 U/L
ALP 288 U/L

108 i. The differential diagnosis given the above history is wide but likely to be infective. The probable diagnosis is hepatitis A infection, although the other hepatotropic viruses (B, C, D, and E) can all cause an acute icteric illness.

ii. In most patients infected with hepatitis A virus the disease runs an uncomplicated course. In the majority of cases, symptoms disappear and aminotransferase activity returns to normal 3–4 weeks after the illness. Fatigability and depression, however, can persist longer. Some patients develop a cholestatic form of the disease. This is characterised by pruritus, fever, diarrhea, weight loss, and bilirubin levels persisting above 9.9 mg/dL (169.3 µmol/L) for a clinical course of at least 12 weeks. This form of the disease has an excellent prognosis although a case can be made for cutting short the jaundice, and relieving the severe itching, with a short course of oral steroids. Although hepatitis A is usually a benign disease of short duration, prolonged abnormalities in biochemical liver tests have been described. Patients who develop protracted clinical and biochemical features of hepatitis A infection interestingly retain the acute serological response to the virus (anti-HAV IgM). Hepatitis A may recur within a few weeks of apparent recovery, even after normalization of liver tests. This second bout may be icteric or anicteric, symptomatic or asymptomatic. In three cases a second relapse of the disease has been observed. Although liver biopsy may show transient features suggesting chronic hepatitis A infection, there are no documented cases of unresolved hepatitis A, or cirrhosis attributable to hepatitis A virus. A rare complication of hepatitis A infection is fulminant hepatic failure. This is characterized by increasing jaundice, deterioration in liver tests, and eventually encephalopathy and death. The mortality of hospitalised patients with hepatitis A infection is <0.2% and seems to correlate with age. The treatment of fulminant hepatitis where prognostic scores predict a fatal outcome is liver transplantation. In patients who survive hepatic coma caused by acute hepatitis A infection there is no evidence of fibrosis or cirrhosis.

109 i. This gross finding shows an enlarged left lobe of the liver secondary to a hepatic adenoma with hemorrhage into the subcapsular space. This tumor also bled into the peritoneum, leading to the death of this patient.

ii. The histologic finding consists of pale staining hepatocytes. An hepatic (or liver cell) adenoma is characterized by swollen hepatocytes, without the usual lobular architecture of portal triads and central veins.

iii. A CT scan would have shown a tumor mass in the left lobe and might have prompted urgent surgery for resection.

iv. This tumor, when presenting as a smaller lesion in an earlier stage, can be confused with focal nodular hyperplasia. After cavernous hemangioma, these tumors are the most common benign tumors of the liver. Hepatic adenomas, but not focal nodular hyperplasia, are related to long term use of oral contraceptives. Moreover, hepatic adenomas may rupture when large (4–6 cm [1.6–2.3 in]), whereas focal nodular hyperplasia has no major risk of rupture. Giant hepatic adenomas may be so large that resection is not possible and liver transplantation is required.

110 A 53-year-old chronic alcoholic with cirrhosis is admitted for alcohol detoxification. Physical examination reveals a pulse of 110 beats/min, blood pressure 150/110 mmHg (20/14.7 kPa), spider angiomata, a small amount of ascites, tremor, and confusion. Laboratory investigations are shown.

Albumin 3.6 g/dL (36 g/L)
Total bilirubin 1.2 mg/dL (20.5 μmol/L)
Prothrombin time 13 seconds

i. What is the differential diagnosis for the patient's confusion?
ii. How can the nature of the patient's shaking tremor help determine the cause of his confusion?
iii. How can the cause of the patient's confusion be determined?

111 A 60-year-old female with a past medical history of psoriasis and noninsulin dependent diabetes mellitus presented to her dermatologist for routine follow-up. She had been taking oral methotrexate 7.5 mg per week for more than 10 years. Physical examination revealed a mildly obese woman with no stigmata of chronic liver disease. The liver was palpable one fingerbreadth below the right costal margin and was 12 cm (4.7 in) in span in the midclavicular line. There was no ascites or splenomegaly. Laboratory studies pre- and 10 years post-methotrexate treatment are shown.
A percutaneous liver biopsy was performed (111).
i. Comment on the liver histology.
ii. What is the most likely diagnosis?
iii. What risk factors in this patient may have increased her likelihood of developing this problem?

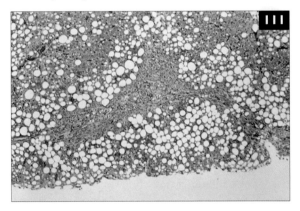

	AST U/L	ALT U/L	Bilirubin mg/dL (μmol/L)	Albumin g/dL (g/L)	Prothrombin time (seconds)
Pre-methotrexate	34	30	0.8 (13.7)	4.0 (40)	11.2
Post-methotrexate	72	52	1.0 (17.1)	3.4 (34)	12.4

110 i. The differential diagnosis would include hepatic encephalopathy associated with cirrhosis, alcohol withdrawal delirium, ethanol neurotoxicity, nutritional deficiency secondary to chronic alcoholism (hypoglycemia, thiamine deficiency, Wernicke– Korsakoff syndrome, pellegra, Marchiafava–Bignami syndrome, and severe hypophosphatemia). Finally, a subdural hematoma from head trauma should also be considered.

ii. Tremor is frequently present in patients with alcohol withdrawal and hepatic encephalopathy. In alcohol withdrawal, a high frequency tremor caused by activity of antagonistic muscles is encountered. It diminishes when the patient is inactive and increases with attempted motor activity and emotional stress. The tremor of hepatic encephalopathy (asterixis), in contrast, is characterized by a biphasic 'flapping' move-ment of the outstretched hands caused by intermittent, muscle contraction in an attempt to maintain posture.

iii. The precise diagnosis of confusion in a patient with decompensated cirrhosis who has been drinking recently is frequently difficult. Hepatic encephalopathy is suggested in a patient who responds to empiric lactulose therapy. Similarly, a response to treatment for alcohol withdrawal or thiamine therapy will indicate the diagnosis. MRI can help distinguish ethanol neurotoxicity from nutritional deficiency as specific macroscopic lesions of Wernicke's encephalopathy, central pontine myelinolysis, cerebellar degeneration, and the Marchiafava–Bignami syndrome can be demonstrated.

111 i. The biopsy shows fatty change in hepatocytes and fibrosis (indicated by the blue-green trichome stain) extending from the portal tracts. A mononuclear infiltrate is also present.

ii. The histology is typical for methotrexate induced hepatotoxicity with fatty change and portal fibrosis.

iii. Cumulative dose, advanced age, obesity, impaired renal function, and diabetes mellitus have all been associated with an increased risk of methotrexate hepato-toxicity. Other putative risk factors include alcohol consumption, Felty's syndrome, and pulmonary fibrosis. Methotrexate hepatotoxicity has received considerable attention over the years. Most of the current concepts of its long term hepatotoxic potential have evolved from its use in nonmalignant diseases, namely, psoriasis and rheumatoid arthritis. The risk of liver histology worsening is significantly greater in patients with psoriasis (33%) than in patients with rheumatoid arthritis (24%). The risk of developing either advanced fibrosis or cirrhosis is also greater in psoriasis patients (7.7% vs 2.7%). Most studies indicate that the incidence of cirrhosis is low with a total cumulative dose below 1.5 g. Liver biopsy is recommended when this dose is exceeded in patients with psoriasis. Cirrhosis attributable to methotrexate treatment may be complicated by portal hypertension and liver failure, but in the majority of patients, the disease is subclinical and nonprogressive. The development of fibrosis and cirrhosis with long term, low dose methotrexate is usually covert, with little evidence of hepatocellular necrosis. Aminotransferase levels are frequently normal and monitoring of biochemical liver tests often fails to alert the physician to the development of significant liver disease. Hepatic fibrosis from methotrexate may regress when therapy with the drug is discontinued.

112 A 6-day-old male presents with jaundice. He is breast feeding well. On physical examination he does not have hepatosplenomegaly. Laboratory investigation reveals a serum total bilirubin level of 17 mg/dL (291 μmol/L), all unconjugated bilirubin.

What is the differential diagnosis?

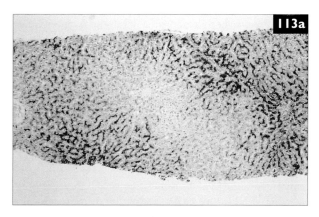

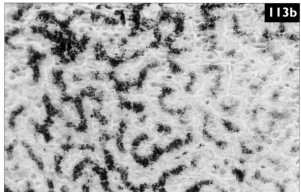

113 There are several different clinical syndromes of iron overload which have characteristic histologic features. Determine the correct syndrome in the case below and the cases in **114**.

A 48-year-old, white male complains of arthralgias and fatigue. Laboratory investigations are shown. A percutaneous liver biopsy is performed and a photomicrograph of the Perls' Prussian blue stain is shown (**113a, b**).

What is the most likely diagnosis?

CBC normal
Biochemical liver test results normal
Fasting transferrin saturation 82%
Serum ferritin 1,280 ng/mL (22.9 μmol/L)

112 Physiologic jaundice of the newborn is a transient benign condition and is the most frequent cause of newborn jaundice. In full term healthy infants it usually peaks on day 3 of life, and resolves during the first week. Physiologic jaundice must be differentiated from pathologic jaundice. Pathologic jaundice may be present if the infant is born jaundiced or if jaundice occurs in the first 24 hours of life, the total bilirubin exceeds 12 mg/dL (205 μmol/L), jaundice persists beyond the first week of life, and if there is a direct hyperbilirubinemia. Physiologic jaundice may result from immaturity of the bilirubin conjugating enzymes (glucuronyl transferase). Other causes contributing to jaundice in the newborn include bilirubin overproduction, delayed cellular transport of bilirubin by immaturity of transport proteins, and enhanced reabsorption of bilirubin caused by the enterohepatic circulation. Bilirubin overproduction may result from ABO and Rh incompatibility resulting in hemolysis of RBCs. Sepsis may cause increased unconjugated bilirubin levels. The presence of a cephalohematoma secondary to a difficult delivery or polycythemia caused by delayed clamping of the umbilical cord can increase RBC mass and contribute to hyper-bilirubinemia. Hereditary RBC membrane defects (spherocytosis, elliptocytosis) and hemoglobinopathies can cause elevated bilirubin levels in infancy. Breast milk jaundice is a benign condition which usually appears between the sixth and eighth days of life in an otherwise healthy breast feeding infant. The etiology of breast milk jaundice remains unknown. Rarer causes of newborn jaundice include Lucey–Driscoll syndrome and Crigler–Najjar syndrome. Lucey–Driscoll syndrome is a rare familial disorder characterized by transient hyperbilirubinemia secondary to an unidentified inhibitor of glucuronyl transferase in the sera of these infants and their mothers. It is not present in breast milk. Crigler–Najjar syndrome is another rare hereditary syndrome in which there is a deficiency of bilirubin glucuronyl transferase, the enzyme system responsible for bilirubin conjugation. Type I is the severe form in which there is no enzyme activity and infants are at risk for the development of kernicterus. Type II Crigler–Najjar patients have a partial deficiency of glucuronyl transferase which is inducible by phenobarbital therapy. Hypothyroidism is also associated with unconjugated hyperbilirubinemia. It is postulated that thyroid hormone deficiency causes a reduction in glucuronyl transferase activity.

113 The pattern of iron deposition is consistent with homozygous hereditary hemochromatosis. The hepatic iron concentration is 13,580 μg/g with a calculated hepatic iron index of 5.05.

Hematocrit 18%
Hemoglobin 6.1 g/dL (61 g/L)
LDH elevated
Total bilirubin 1.8 mg/dL
  (30.78 µmol/L)
AST 58 U/l
ALT normal
ALP normal
Albumin normal
Fasting transferrin saturation 78%
Serum ferritin 1,280 ng/mL
  (22.9 µmol/L)

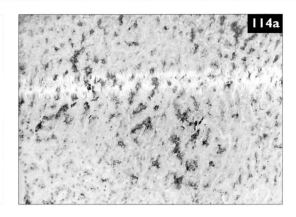

114 There are several different clinical syndromes of iron overload which have characteristic histologic features. Determine the correct syndrome in the case in **113** and the cases below.

i. A 48-year-old, white male was seen for evaluation of abnormal biochemical liver test results. He admits to drinking more than a six-pack of beer per night and has done so for many years. Physical examination shows hepatomegaly. Laboratory data show macrocytosis with a MCV of 105 fL and modest thrombocytopenia with a platelet count of 110,000/mm^3 (110 × 10^9/L). Other laboratory investigations are shown above. A percutaneous liver biopsy is performed and the Perls' Prussian blue stain is shown (**114a**). What is the most likely diagnosis?

ii. A 48-year-old, white male has a 3-year history of severe toxin-induced acquired aplastic anemia. Over the past 3 years, he has received 80 units of packed red cells to correct his anemia. Laboratory investigations are shown below. The Perls' Prussian blue stain of his percutaneous liver biopsy is shown (**114b**). How would you characterize his biopsy?

AST 165 U/L
ALT 68 U/L
ALP 140 U/L
Total bilirubin 1.5 mg/dL
  (25.6 µmol/L)
Serum albumin 3.3 g/dL (33 g/L)
Fasting transferrin saturation 78%
Serum ferritin level 1,280 ng/mL
  (22.9 µmol/L)

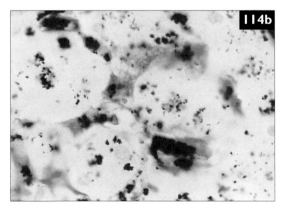

114 i. The deposition of iron is panlobular and is both in Kupffer cells and in hepatocytes. There is only a mild increase in iron stores. This is compatible with secondary iron overload associated with alcoholic liver disease. The hepatic iron concentration is 1,600 µg/g with a calculated hepatic iron index of 0.59.

ii. The histologic pattern of iron deposition is panlobular with a marked increase in iron deposition in Kupffer cells as well as in hepatocytes. This is consistent with the pattern seen in transfusional iron overload. The hepatic iron concentration is 15,280 µg/g. The hepatic iron index is not calculated in transfusional iron overload.

These three examples of clinical cases (**113, 114**) with abnormal iron studies illustrate the major three disorders of iron metabolism: hereditary hemochromatosis, secondary iron overload caused by chronic liver disease, and transfusional iron overload. The other two main categories of iron storage disease are neonatal iron overload and African iron overload. It is important to understand these various distinctions and to describe and categorize patients appropriately as diagnostic work-up and decisions about therapy differ for the various disorders. Hereditary hemochromatosis should be the term reserved for the single gene (HFE) on chromosome 6 disorder in which there is an increase in gastrointestinal absorption of dietary iron. The hepatic distribution of iron in homozygous hereditary hemochromatosis is periportal and predominantly parenchymal (hepato-cellular). In secondary iron overload, there is an increase in iron absorption stimulated by some process other than in hereditary hemochromatosis. The iron-loading is usually mild to moderate with iron deposition in Kupffer cells as well as parenchymal cells often in a lobular distribution rather than a periportal distribution. In transfusional iron overload the iron burden is derived from transfused RBCs that have been phagocytized by cells of the reticuloendothelial system (Kupffer cells in the liver). Thus, the iron burden is dependent on the number of tranfusions that have occurred. The hepatic distribution of iron is predominantly in Kupffer cells and is usually in a panlobular distribution. In the first patient (**113**), the hepatic iron concentration and calculated hepatic iron index, along with the hepatic distribution of iron, are entirely consistent with homozygous hereditary hemochromatosis. His HFE gene status should be checked. This patient should be treated with therapeutic phlebotomy until his iron stores are depleted and his first-degree relatives should be screened with fasting transferin saturation and ferritin levels to rule out hemo-chromatosis. The second patient has alcoholic liver disease which is suggested by his clinical history of excess alcohol ingestion, his macrocytosis, and his pattern of liver enzyme abnormalities with an AST higher than an ALT. His hepatic iron concentration is only slightly increased, consistent with mild secondary iron overload. The hepatic iron distribution is panlobular, in both hepatocytes and Kupffer cells, typical for this disorder. His treatment should consist of adequate nutrition and abstinence from alcohol. He does not require treatment to remove hepatic iron. The third patient has transfusional iron overload which is discerned by his history of having received numerous RBC transfusions. The histologic findings of iron predominantly in Kupffer cells are characteristic. This patient cannot be treated by phlebotomy and should be treated with deferoxamine given either as a continuous subcutaneous infusion or a night-time intravenous infusion.

Patients with all three of these disorders can have identical blood iron studies, indicating the inability to distinguish these syndromes without a liver biopsy.

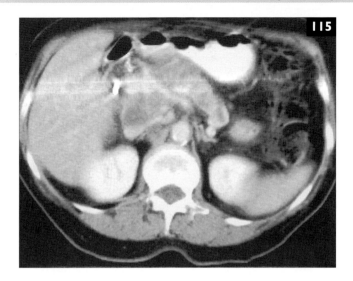

115 A 74-year-old female presents with obstructive jaundice and a large upper abdominal mass. An ERCP fails because of the presence of a large obstructing and ulcerating lesion in the second part of the duodenum. A large amount of tenacious mucus is seen. A CT scan is performed following endoscopy (**115**).
i. What does the CT scan show?
ii. What is the most likely diagnosis and the differential diagnosis?
iii. What is the prognosis?

116 A 59-year-old male was brought to the emergency room with severe vomiting and inability to stand. An empty bottle of acetaminophen (paracetamol) and a half-empty bottle of whisky were found at the bedside by a relative. The patient had a long history of depression and made a suicide attempt 2 years previously. The emergency room physicians suspected acetaminophen overdose and implemented an emergency diagnostic work-up and treatment including intravenous access, determination of acetaminophen level, stomach lavage, and therapy with N-acetyl cysteine.
i. How does the liver metabolize acetaminophen?
ii. Are chronic alcoholics at an increased risk for acetaminophen hepatotoxicity?
iii. How does N-acetyl cysteine alter the course of acetaminophen hepatotoxicity?

115 i. The CT scan shows a cystic mass occupying the head of the pancreas associated with dilation of the main pancreatic duct. A stent is seen within the common bile duct.

ii. The differential diagnosis of cystic masses within the pancreas includes neoplastic and inflammatory diseases. The most benign neoplasm is a cystadenoma and these may produce either serous or mucinous fluid. More commonly a cystadenocarcinoma occurs. This tends to occur in women and occupies the head of the gland. Occasionally ductal pancreatic cancers may exhibit cystic change. Cystic change within the pancreas can follow attacks of acute pancreatitis or be a feature of chronic pancreatitis. In this case the large abdominal mass with production of a large volume of mucus is suggestive of a cystadenocarcinoma. This was proven on biopsy.

iii. Unlike cancers arising from the pancreatic duct which have a dismal prognosis, the prognosis of cystadenocarcinoma is relatively good. Tumors tend to be slowly growing and treatment is based upon alleviation of biliary obstruction. Removal of the tumor by a Whipple's operation may be curative. The 5 year survival rate is around 50% compared with 1–2% for adenocarcinoma of the pancreas.

116 i. Acetaminophen is oxidized via cytochrome P450 enzymes and conjugated with glutathione.

ii. Yes. See the explanation below.

iii. By providing the amino acid cysteine, glutathione synthesis is enhanced. Glutathione is pivotal in the conjugation of the toxic metabolite of acetaminophen to a benign derivative. One of the physiological properties of the liver is the metabolism of drugs. The processes used by the liver to detoxify xenobiotics include reduction, oxidation, conjugation, and hydrolysis. Clinically, nausea and vomiting characterize the clinical presentation of acute acetaminophen-induced hepatotoxicity, accompanied by marked elevation of aminotransferase activities and bilirubin. This can be followed by acute liver failure. Acetaminophen intake in the order of 10 g is associated with hepatotoxicity. Immediate treatment with N-acetyl cysteine is required (preferably within 12 hours of the overdose). However, even when the overdose has been estimated to occur more than 12 hours before the encounter with the patient, treatment with N-acetyl cysteine is recommended. Understanding the mechanism of acetaminophen hepatotoxicity has facilitated the application of effective therapy within a specific therapeutic window. Acetaminophen is oxidized via cytochrome P450 enzymes to N-acetyl-p-benzoquinoneimine (NAPQI) which is the major metabolite responsible for the hepatotoxicity of this drug. Under normal conditions, NAPQI is conjugated with glutathione and excreted in the urine. In conditions associated with glutathione depletion, NAPQI accumulates. Binding of NAPQI to mitochondria of hepatocytes is implicated in the pathogenesis of this injury. Individuals taking substances that induce cytochrome P450 enzymes such as those who drink alcohol in excess or are under treatment with phenobarbital, produce more NAPQI and are at increased risk for toxicity. In addition, glutathione depletion, such as that associated with excess intake of alcohol, is also associated with an increased risk of acetaminophen hepatotoxicity.

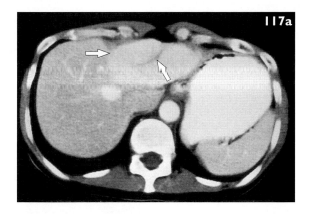

117 A 38-year-old female presented for an evaluation for gallstones. She had a long history of dyspepsia with postprandial upper abdominal discomfort. Percutaneous ultrasound examination of the abdomen revealed a well defined solid mass in the liver. There were no gallstones. Blood tests showed normal biochemical liver tests, nonreactive HBsAg, anti-HBc, anti-HCV, antinuclear, antismooth muscle, and anti-mitochondrial antibodies. Serum alphafetoprotein and ferritin were within normal range. Review of medical history revealed no alcohol abuse or oral contraceptive use. A CT scan of the abdomen showed a solitary mass with irregular borders and a central cleft (**117a**, arrows).

i. Will you inform this patient that she has a malignant liver tumor?
ii. What tests would you order to obtain a definitive diagnosis in this patient?
iii. Would you refer this patient for hepatic resection?

118 A 43-year-old male with a past history of increased ethanol consumption and a remote history of intravenous drug abuse is found to have cirrhosis on a liver biopsy performed to evaluate abnormal biochemical liver test results, which are shown. An anti-HCV is positive by ELISA and a

Total bilirubin 1.5 mg/dL (25 μmol/L)
AST 90 U/L
ALT 65 U/L
Serum albumin 3.2 g/dL (32 g/L)
Prothrombin time 12.2 seconds

hepatitis C virus-RNA assay result is 5,200,000 genomes/mL. On examination, he is found to be an alert male with no peripheral stigmata of chronic liver disease. His liver span is 14 cm (5.5 in) in the midclavicular line by percussion and his liver edge is firm, slightly nodular, and is palpable 5 cm (1.9 in) below the right costal margin. His spleen is palpable 3 cm (1.2 in) below the left costal margin. He has no detectable ascites. A screening endoscopy reveals two chains of large esophageal varices. The patient is now abstinent, is determined to change his life style, and has found a regular job.

What is this patient's risk of experiencing an episode of esophageal variceal hemorrhage in the next 2–3 years?

117 i. No. The CT scan is consistent with a malignant or a benign hepatic tumor. The liver parenchyma is homogeneous and the liver and spleen sizes normal. No underlying liver disease is suggested by CT and biochemical liver tests. Risk factors for hepatocellular carcinoma (viral infection, alcohol abuse, autoimmune hepatitis, hemochromatosis, and long term oral contraceptives) are absent. Serum alphafetoprotein is normal. However, up to 30% of patients with hepatocellular carcinoma have normal serum alphafetoprotein. A benign hepatic neoplasm should be considered. Common benign tumors include hepatocellular adenoma, focal nodular hyperplasia, hemangioma, and hepatic cysts. In patients with cir-

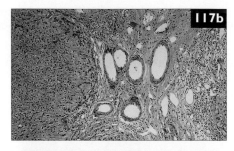

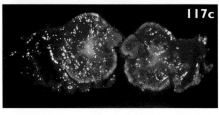

rhosis, benign regenerative nodules often mimic hepatocellular carcinoma. A central scar suggests a diagnosis of focal nodular hyperplasia.

ii. Biopsy of the lesion may be helpful in diagnosis. Focal nodular hyperplasia is suggested by the central scar with relatively large blood vessels (117b).

iii. Hepatic resection is not necessary if the benign nature of a lesion can be determined by imaging studies or biopsy. In some cases, this can only be accomplished by resection (117c). Benign hepatic tumors do not require surgical resection except under the following circumstances: high risk of rupture and hemorrhage seen in large hemangiomas (more than 10 cm [3.9 in]), and adenomas with a prior history of pain (indicating intratumoral hemorrhage); planned pregnancy, which may increase the risk for hemorrhage because of increase in tumor size; and the risk of transformation from hepatocellular adenomas to carcinomas, which should be considered for large adenomas. Estrogenic hormones should be discontinued in patients with these benign neoplasms, particularly heptocellular adenomas, and may result in tumor regression.

118 This patient has a 25–33% chance of experiencing an episode of esophageal variceal hemorrhage in the next 2–3 years. Prospective studies of patients with cirrhosis and large esophageal varices have demonstrated a 25–33% risk of initial variceal hemorrhage over 3 years. The highest risk period for bleeding is within the initial year of the diagnosis of esophageal varices with the risk diminishing in succeeding years. Risk factors for initial variceal hemorrhage include their size, presence of endoscopically determined red color signs (e.g. red weal signs, hemocystic spots), and estimates of the severity of liver disease (Child's classification). Active alcohol consumption is a risk factor for patients with alcoholic liver disease. Nonselective beta blockers (propranalol, nadolol) have been shown to reduce the chances of variceal bleeding. Prophylactic variceal sclerotherapy or banding has not been demonstrated to affect mortality. Further trials of banding are in progress.

119 A 62-year-old chronic alcoholic male with a history of repeated attacks of gout is admitted for alcohol detoxification. Routine laboratory tests reveal a serum uric acid level of 11.2 mg/dL (0.7 mmol/L). Features of his physical examination are demonstrated (119 a, b).

i. Comment on the features found on physical examination.

ii. What is the relationship between the patient's alcoholism and gout?

iii. What is the mechanism for this interaction?

iv. How can this relationship be proven in this patient?

v. What other metabolic effects are associated with chronic alcoholism?

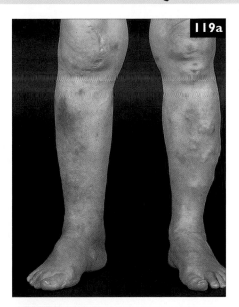

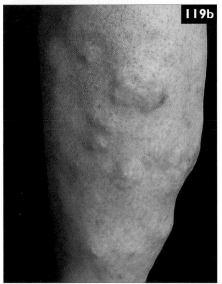

119 i. Tophaceous gout with multiple subcutaneous deposits of yellowish white excrescences are present in the lower extremities. Severe gouty arthritis is also seen.

ii. The consumption of large amounts of alcoholic beverages is a common predisposing or precipitating cause of gout.

iii. During the oxidation of ethanol to acetaldehyde and then acetate, hydrogen is transferred to the cofactor nicotinamide adenine dinucleotide (NAD), converting it to the reduced form NADH. The generation of large amounts of these reducing equivalents overwhelms the ability of the hepatocyte to maintain redox homeostasis. The enhanced NADH/NAD ratio is reflected by an increased lactate/pyruvate ratio and hyperlactacidemia from decreased utilization and enhanced production of lactate by the liver. The hyperlactacidemia and the alcohol-induced ketosis, in turn reduce the capacity of the kidney to excrete uric acid, leading to secondary hyperuricemia. Increased acetate levels also enhance ATP breakdown and purine generation and further promote hyperuricemia.

iv. Repeat the serum uric acid level. Within 3–6 days of abstinence, the serum acid level frequently declines by over 50%.

v. Hypoglycemia may develop in subjects with glycogen stores depleted by starvation in whom hepatic gluconeogenesis is blocked as a consequence of the increased NADH/NAD ratio. Conversely, glucose intolerance resulting from decreased peripheral glucose utilization may also develop. Fatty liver (steatosis) is a common consequence of chronic alcoholism. It also results from the increased NADH/NAD ratio which promotes hepatic triglyceride accumulation. In addition, fatty acid oxidation is decreased. Hyperlipemia, which involves all lipoprotein classes is commonly present. Ketonemia and, in extreme situations, alcoholic ketoacidosis may develop in subjects in whom an increased fat load on the liver is combined with a relative depletion of hepatic carbohydrate intermediates necessary for the oxidation of fat through the citric acid cycle. The effect of alcohol on ketogenesis is most predominant in the fasting state when alcohol has disappeared from the blood and preferentially involves increases in beta-hydroxybutyrate. This is not readily detected with the usual laboratory tests for ketones that use the nitroprusside reaction. As a result, the complication is frequently overlooked. Alcoholic ketoacidosis typically develops in subjects who have a recent history of increased alcohol consumption which is followed by anorexia, hyperemesis, and cessation of food and alcohol. Ketoacidosis usually occurs within 40 hours or more after the last intake of alcohol at which time the patient presents with starvation, progressive dehydration, and mild mental confusion. Blood glucose levels on admission are variable. Acidosis is frequently present with beta-hydroxybutyrate levels as high as 20 mM. Clinical improvement occurs rapidly in response to intravenous glucose and saline with the ketosis usually disappearing within 12–18 hours.

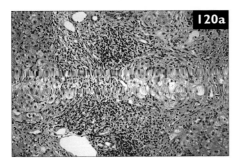

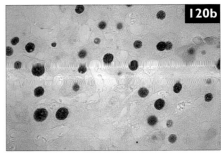

120 A patient survived the acute phase of hepatitis D (see **66**), became asymptomatic, and 20 months after the acute episode was readmitted. Laboratory investigations and immunohistochemistry results are shown. Ultrasound imaging revealed a moderate liver enlargement with nonhomogenous structure and no signs of portal hypertension. Liver biopsy showed a chronic active hepatitis (**120a**).

The patient was treated with alpha-2b recombinant interferon at 10 MU three times a week for 12 months. During treatment ALT serum levels became normal, hepatitis D virus-RNA, hepatitis B virus-DNA and HBeAg were cleared from serum. IgM anti-HD decreased to a titer of 10^{-3}. HBsAg remained positive. After stopping interferon, ALT returned to pretreatment levels, followed by an increase in IgM titer to 10^{-5}, hepatitis D virus-RNA persisted negative (**120c**).

i. Was the patient a good candidate for interferon treatment ?

ii. Was the interferon schedule adequate?

iii. Which is the best test to monitor the efficacy of interferon treatment ?

iv. After the interferon failure, what alternative treatment, if any, would you suggest?

v. Was the interferon treatment worthwhile ?

AST 128 U/L
ALT 158 U/L
Prothrombin time 45 seconds
Albumin 4.2 g/dL (42 g/L)
Hemoglobin 14.5 g/dL (145 g/L)
WBC count 9,400/mm³ (9.4 × 10⁹/L)
Platelet count 183,000/mm³ (183 × 10⁹/L)
HBsAg present, IgM anti-HBc absent, HBeAg present, hepatitis B virus-DNA present
Anti-HD present, IgM anti-HD present (titer 10^{-4}), hepatitis D virus-RNA present
Anti-HCV absent
Anti-liver–kidney microsomal antibodies present

Immunohistochemistry results were:
Hepatitis D antigen nuclear diffuse (**120b**)
HBcAg nuclear focal
HBsAg positive cytoplasmic

120 i. In chronic hepatitis D no factors predictive of response to interferon have been identified with the possible exception of a short duration of hepatitis D virus disease. The best results have been reported in former drug addicts likely to have recently acquired hepatitis B and D virus infections. A concomitant HIV infection, if immunocompetence is preserved, does not influence the likelihood of response. The presence of anti-liver-kidney microsomal autoantibodies, frequently detectable in chronic hepatitis D, has not been reported to be significantly associated with interferon triggered autoimmune phenomena. The patient was, therefore, an optimal candidate for interferon treatment. He did respond from the virological and biochemical point of view, but response did not outlast the end of treatment. The result is not surprising as in chronic hepatitis D long term response to interferon is under 10%.

ii. Several schedules of interferon have been tried but the most safe and efficacious is the one employed in this patient: alpha-2 recombinant interferon 9–10 MU thrice weekly for 1 year. Administration of higher doses or more prolonged treatment periods do not grant higher rates of long term response and yield a high risk of severe psychiatric side effects principally in the form of severe depression, occasionally leading to suicide.

iii. The patient was monitored with markers for hepatitis B and D virus infection and replication. Serum hepatitis D virus-RNA became negative during treatment and persisted negative when interferon treatment ceased. Nonetheless, the disease recurred. The clearance of hepatitis D virus-RNA, if associated with normal ALT levels, is therefore a good marker of interferon efficacy but is not able to predict long term response. Long term response is associated in more than 90% of cases to the clearance of IgM anti-HD and HBsAg from serum. In this patient both markers remained positive.

iv. No alternative treatment to interferon is available at present. Therapeutic attempts with ribavirin and thymosin derivatives gave no significant therapeutic benefit.

v. Although the patient was not cured by interferon, the treatment has to be regarded as worthwhile. During treatment active hepatitis B virus (HBeAg and hepatitis D virus-DNA) and hepatitis D virus replication (hepatitis D virus-RNA) became undetectable. Both events have been shown to be associated with reduced severity and progression of hepatitis D disease.

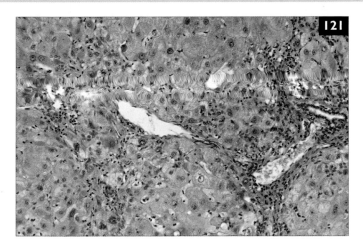

121 A 28 year old male presented with an initial episode of 'acute hepatitis' 8 years previously. Serologic studies to exclude viral hepatitis were negative and a hepatic biopsy was obtained (121). A diagnosis of chronic active hepatitis was made on the basis of histology showing inflammatory cell infiltrates, piecemeal necrosis, and bridging fibrosis. A trial of steroid therapy resulted in no improvement. Over the next several years the patient noted some tremulousness and more recently, difficulty with his speech. Examination showed decreased liver span, splenomegaly, mild tremors, and dysarthria. Laboratory investigations are shown.

Hemoglobin 14 g/dL (140 g/L)
Platelet count 71,000/mm^3 (71 × 10^9/L)
Prothrombin time 15 seconds
ALT 206 U/L
AST 60 U/L
Total bilirubin 0.9 mg/dL (15.4 µmol/L)
ALP 90 U/L
Albumin3.6 g/dL (36 g/L)
Monospot negative
Alpha-1-antitrypsin normal
Ferritin 350 ng/mL (7.0 µmol/l)
Transferrin saturation 24%
Autoantibodies absent

i. What diagnosis must be considered? What tests should be obtained?
ii. What treatment should be initiated?

122 A 45-year-old male patient has multiple symptoms associated with hereditary hemochromatosis. He has begun weekly phlebotomy.
i. Which of his symptoms are expected to improve?
ii. What will happen to his liver disease?
iii. What studies should be offered to his family?

121 i. The differential diagnosis of chronic active hepatitis includes many possibilities such as drug induced liver disease, viral hepatitis, immune mediated hepatitis, and metabolic disease. The development of neurologic symptoms in association with liver disease should initiate investigations to exclude Wilson's disease. These studies should include a slit-lamp examination for the presence of Kayser–Fleischer rings, a serum ceruloplasmin, 24 hour urinary copper excretion after penicillamine, liver biopsy for histology, and quantitative copper determination. A slit-lamp examination of this patient revealed the presence of Kayser–Fleischer rings. His serum ceruloplasmin was found to be 150 mg/L (normal 200–400 mg/L). Urinary copper excretion was also found to be 390 µg/24 hours (normal 40 µg/24 hours). On the basis of these data a diagnosis of Wilson's disease was established, even without a quantitative hepatic copper determination. If Kayser–Fleischer rings were not present, a repeat biopsy for quantitative copper determination would have been appropriate.
ii. Specific treatment for Wilson's disease was initiated with the copper chelator penicillamine. A repeat 24 hour urine for copper showed more than 4 mg/24 hours. The serum transaminase activities, albumin and prothrombin time returned to normal after 6 months. Minimal residual neurologic symptoms persisted.

122 i. Typical symptoms associated with hereditary hemochromatosis that improve with treatment include fatigue, malaise, and right upper quadrant abdominal pain. Arthralgias, arthritis, and impotence typically do not improve with phlebotomy therapy. Cardiac manifestations can improve. Those patients who are diabetic can be more easily managed once they have become iron depleted. Skin pigmentation is reduced with phlebotomy therapy. If biochemical liver tests are abnormal because of iron overload, with reduction in hepatic iron stores, these will return to normal.
ii. Established cirrhosis is not likely to improve, but about 30% of patients with increased fibrosis can have some reduction in fibrosis.
iii. All first-degree relatives should be screened with fasting transferrin saturation and ferritin levels. Genetic testing for the HFE gene should be reserved for siblings. One must remember that whenever a patient with hereditary hemochromatosis is identified, the physician's responsibility is not only to the patient but to his or her family as this is an inherited disorder. The physician should advise the patient to identify all first-degree relatives to be screened for hemochromatosis. Screening should consist of fasting transferrin saturation and ferritin levels. In individuals over 40 years of age or those with abnormal liver test results, if either of these is abnormal, a liver biopsy should be obtained for routine histology including iron stains, determination of hepatic iron concentration, and calculation of hepatic iron index. For individuals <40 years of age, if these values are normal, they should be repeated again in 2–3 years. For individuals >40 years of age with normal iron studies, there is a <3% chance that they will have homozygous hemochromatosis.

123 A 3-month-old female presents to the emergency room with a 2 day history of an upper respiratory infection, anorexia, vomiting, and irritability. The girl is breast fed. She is admitted to the hospital for intravenous fluid administration. Within hours, she has developed hepatomegaly, ascites, anasarca, and bleeding.

Total bilirubin 1.2 mg/dL (20.5 μmol/L)
AST 60 U/L
ALT 55 U/L
Prothrombin time 17 seconds
Partial thromboplastin time 45 seconds

Some nurses have noted that the patient is emitting a peculiar odor of boiled cabbage. Laboratory investigations are shown. Family history is positive for a sibling who died from an 'unknown' liver disorder presumed metabolic at 6 months of age.
i. What is the differential diagnosis?
ii. What additional laboratory studies would you order?

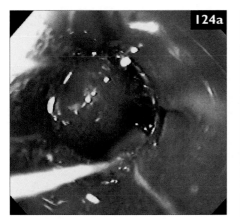
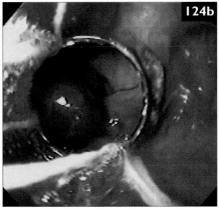

124 The gastroenterologist is called to the emergency room to evaluate a patient with melena and suspected liver disease. The endoscopist finds large esophageal varices with stigmata of recent hemorrhage, a mild portal hypertensive gastropathy, and no other potential source of bleeding. The endoscopic view of the esophagus shows a distended varix at the end of the band ligator endoscope (124a). This varix has had a band placed which preserves the polpyoid nature of the varix (124b) until the ischemic tissue sloughs. Why was this therapy chosen?

123 i. Several inborn errors of metabolism have similar clinical manifestations within days to weeks after birth. Hepatosplenomegaly, jaundice, bleeding, vomiting, and failure to thrive may be prominent. These include galactosemia, hereditary fructose intolerance, and tyrosinemia. The diagnosis should be suspected because of the positive family history. Liver disease associated with cataracts and psychomotor retardation suggests a diagnosis of galactosemia in a breast fed infant or infant receiving a lactose containing formula. A history of vomiting, aversion to sweet foods, failure to thrive, and fructosuria would suggest a diagnosis of hereditary fructose intolerance. Tyrosinemia must be considered in any child with evidence of hepatocellular necrosis, cirrhosis, and abnormal coagulation studies for which a cause is not readily evident. The peculiar odor of boiled cabbage is observed in some patients with tyrosinemia during a hepatic crisis.

ii. Initial screening tests would include urine for nonglucose reducing sugars (i.e. fructose), organic acids, and amino acids. Extreme elevations in serum alpha-feto-protein are more common with tyrosinemia. All forms of liver failure including all three of the above diagnoses may have elevated serum tyrosine and methionine levels, so hypertyrosinemia can not distinguish between the diagnoses. The presence of succinylacetone in serum or urine is pathognomonic for tyrosinemia.

124 For the past 20 years, sclerotherapy has been the preferred treatment to control acute esophageal variceal hemorrhage. More recently, many endoscopists have switched to using esophageal variceal ligation or banding because the side effects are fewer and the efficacy is comparable to sclerotherapy. For patients in whom the bleeding source is gastric varices more than 2–3 cm (0.8–1.2 in) below the esophago-gastric junction or portal hypertensive gastropathy, endoscopic therapy is not indicated. Although a number of randomized controlled trials have compared endo-scopic variceal ligation with sclerotherapy for the prevention of recurrent variceal bleeding, none have specifically been designed to compare efficacy for the control of acute variceal hemorrhage. Nevertheless, a subset analysis of these trials demonstrated that the two techniques are equally effective in controlling the acute bleeding episode. Sclerotherapy is often easier to perform in the acutely bleeding patient. Variceal ligation might be preferred in the patient with stigmata of recent hemorrhage but minimal bleeding at the time of endoscopy. For patients with gastric varices well below the esophagogastric junction or portal hypertensive gastropathy as the source of bleeding, pharmacologic agents such as terlipressin (Glypressin) and the somatostatin analogue, octreotide, are the only established medical therapy for control of bleeding. Pharmacologic and, or, endoscopic therapy is successful in controlling bleeding in 75–90% of patients. For failures of medical therapy, a TIPS is the currently accepted treatment of choice. However, in selected patients with good hepatic reserve (Child's A) and, or, patients who have had several episodes of variceal bleeding, a surgically created shunt, either total or selective, may be preferable to a TIPS procedure.

125 A 32-year-old white male was hospitalized with a sore throat, fever, abdominal pain, nausea, and malaise of 2 weeks duration. His past history included recent onset of a seizure disorder following head trauma, for which he had been receiving phenytoin 400 mg/day for 6 weeks. The patient denied previous blood transfusions, and there was no significant history of drug or alcohol use. His family history was unremarkable for inheritable or infectious diseases. Physical examination revealed an unwell thin man with oral temperature of 100°F (37.8°C). He had a diffuse maculopapular rash with non-tender, mobile cervical lymphadenopathy. The heart and lungs appeared normal. The liver measured 12 cm (4.7 in) in the right midclavicular line and was not tender on palpation. The spleen was palpable on deep inspiration. There was no abdominal tenderness. The remainder of the physical examination was unremarkable. Laboratory investigations are shown. A percutaneous liver biopsy was performed (125a, b).

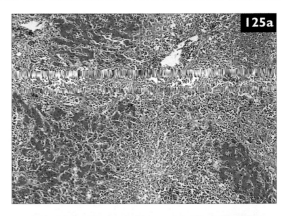

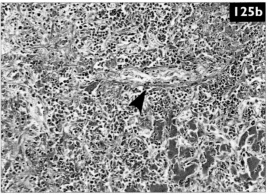

WBC count 19,000/mm³ (19 × 10⁹/L)
WBC differential count 50% neutrophils, 25% lymphocytes, 20% eosinophils, and 5% atypical lymphocytes
AST 174 U/L
ALT 235 IU/L
ALP 329 U/L
Serum albumin, bilirubin, and total protein normal
A monospot test and serologic studies for hepatitis A, B, and C, Epstein–Barr virus, and CMV negative

i. Comment on the liver histology.
ii. What is the most likely diagnosis?
iii. What is the management of this clinical condition?
iv. What is the pathogenesis of this clinical illness?

125 i. 125a shows submassive bridging necrosis and intense mononuclear infiltrates mimicking severe, acute viral hepatitis. The higher magnification of **125b** with a collagen (trichrome) stain shows extensive necrosis most prominent in the centrilobular zone (a residual central vein is indicated by the arrow).

ii. Phenytoin induced allergic hepatitis is the likely diagnosis. This drug induced hypersensitivity syndrome results in a mononucleosis-like illness that may be confused with a viral illness or streptococcal pharyngitis. The danger in this is that the drug is not appropriately withdrawn, despite signs of developing hepatitis.

iii. As with any therapeutic agent, rapid recognition of a possible toxic drug reaction and discontinuation of the drug are fundamental to limiting hepatic damage. Corticosteroids have been employed in a number of instances. They may improve the systemic, serum sickness-like features of the illness, but there is no evidence that they may influence the course of the hepatic lesion or survival.

iv. There are several hypotheses proposed for the mechanism of phenytoin induced liver injury. Many of the symptoms, signs, and laboratory features offer support for the view that phenytoin induced injury is a manifestation of the drug hypersensitivity. In support of this view is the occurrence of pseudomononucleosis syndrome characterized by lymphadenopathy, lymphocytosis, and circulating atypical lymphocytes with additional clinical features of a serum sickness-like illness suggesting the presence of circulating immune complexes. Evidence also exists, however, that phenytoin induced liver injury results from the effects of a toxic intermediary metabolite. Phenytoin is metabolized by the cytochrome P450 system with production of highly reactive arene oxide intermediates. These intermediates are further metabolized to nontoxic metabolites by the enzyme epoxide hydrolase. In the case of either excessive production of phenytoin arene oxides or insufficient metabolism of these metabolites by epoxide hydrolase, they appear to bind covalently to tissue macromolecules. This either leads directly to cellular injury, or results in the production of protein adducts. These act as neoantigens that are ultimately expressed on the cell plasma membrane where they become the targets of immune-mediated cell damage. Available evidence has pointed to an inherited deficiency in epoxide hydrolase activity in patients with phenytoin induced hepatic injury and in their close relatives. These observations suggest that susceptibility to phenytoin induced liver injury is largely determined by genetic factors. The prognosis for reported cases of phenytoin induced hepatic injury has been poor with a case fatality rate of about 30%. Development of chronic hepatitis or cirrhosis in survivors has not been reported.

126 A 64-year-old male presents with a 5 year history of recurrent attacks of cholangitis treated by recurrent courses of antibiotics. There is a previous history of cholecystectomy 20 years earlier.
i. What does the ERCP show?
ii. What is the differential diagnosis?
iii. What is the treatment?

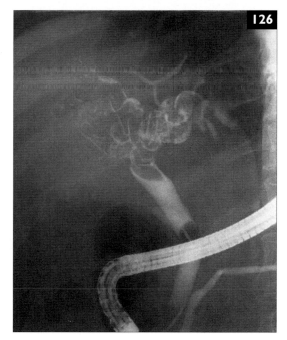

127 A 50-year-old male cirrhotic patient with ascites is being evaluated for liver transplantation. The patient, a former alcoholic, gave up drinking 6 years ago, when the diagnosis of cirrhosis was made. Since then, the only decompensation of his illness has been ascites, which the patient controls with low-sodium diet and 80 mg furosemide and 200 mg spironolactone. He is well nourished. On examination moderate ascites is noted, without ankle edema. An upper endoscopic examination and abdominal ultrasonography and normal serum alphafetoprotein rule out significant esophageal varices and hepatocellular carcinoma, respectively. Laboratory investigations are shown.

Hemoglobin 11 g/dL (110 g/L)
WBC count 2,400/mm³ (2.4 × 10⁹/L)
Platelet count 90,000/mm³ (90 × 10⁹/L)
Bilirubin 2.3 mg/dL (39 μmol/L)
Prothrombin time 21 seconds
Albumin 3.2 g/dL (32 g/L)
Sodium (plasma) 132 mEq/L (132 mmol/L)
Sodium (urine) 11 mEq/day (11 mmol/L)
Potassium 4.3 mEq/L (4.3 mmol/L)
BUN 22 mg/dL (urea 3.65 mmol/L)
Creatinine 0.8 mg/dL (70.72 μmol/L)
Creatinine clearance 85 mL/min
Free water clearance 3 mL/min

i. Which are the variables with the greatest prognostic value in this patient?
ii. Should this patient be included on a liver transplantation waiting list at this time?

126 i. Multiple filling defects are seen throughout the intrahepatic biliary tree. A biliary sphincterotomy had previously been performed and, therefore, cholangiography required inflation of a balloon (seen just above the endoscope). Without occluding the bile duct contrast would have refluxed back into the duodenum and the intrahepatic biliary tree would not have been adequately seen.

ii. The differential diagnosis includes a cholangiocarcinoma but this is unlikely in view of the chronicity of the symptoms. Cholangiocarcinomas may occasionally be polypoid although biliary strictures are more common. Hemobilia following hepatic trauma may have the same appearance. In this case the chronicity of the findings and the history does not support this possibility. This patient has biliary papillomatosis. This is a rare condition in which multiple adenomas exist usually within the intrahepatic biliary tree. Patients present with recurrent cholangitis. This patient also had episodes of biliary obstruction caused by calculi. The adenomas have the potential for malignant transformation.

iii. The treatment of choice is to resect the abnormal area both to prevent recurrent attacks of cholangitis and subsequent malignant change. In a patient with extensive intrahepatic disease such as described here this would necessitate hepatic transplantation.

127 i. In cirrhotic patients with ascites the best predictors of survival are those parameters that reflect the hemodynamic disturbances characteristic of these patients. Thus, mean arterial pressure, plasma and urinary sodium, and parameters of renal function seem to be more reliable than, for example, the Child's–Pugh grade.

ii. The best time to include a cirrhotic patient with ascites in a transplantation program is a difficult issue. It is particularly difficult in this case as there is no evidence of other decompensation such as spontaneous bacterial peritonitis, recurrent variceal bleeding, severe malnutrition, greatly altered hepatocellular function, or encephalopathy. Standard parameters used to estimate liver function, such as the Child's–Pugh classification, are often unreliable in predicting the survival of these patients. On the contrary, variables estimating systemic hemodynamics and renal function are the best predictors.

Thus the appearance of renal failure, significant dilutional hyponatremia or severely decreased mean arterial pressure predict a poor survival and make transplantation advisable. On the other hand, patients able to excrete significant amounts of sodium have a good prognosis so that transplantation may be delayed.

Those cirrhotic patients with ascites who, in the absence of hyponatremia or renal failure, show severe renal sodium reabsorption, make up a large group in which the decision is particularly controversial. Recent reports demonstrate that in these patients, the disturbance of the renal ability to excrete water (estimated through the free water clearance), may be of great help. A compromised free water clearance (defined as <6 mL/min) in spite of other parameters, predicts a poor survival.

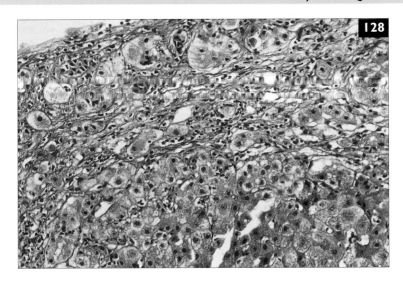

128 A 19-year-old patient with chronic biochemical liver test abnormalities, elevated gammaglobulin levels and a positive antinuclear antibody test underwent a liver biopsy (128).
i. Comment on the pathologic findings.
ii. What is the pathogenesis and natural history of this condition?
iii. What diseases are associated with this condition?
iv. What are the treatment options for this patient?

129 The patient in 85 is now in complete remission on azathioprine 50 mg/day and prednisolone 7.5 mg.
i. Which of the following is true regarding her long term outlook?
A She has a 50% chance of being alive in 5 years time.
B She has a better than 90% of being alive in 10 years.
ii. Should she avoid pregnancy and how should drug therapy be managed?

128, 129: Answers

128 i. The liver biopsy shows architectural distortion with excess fibrosis and portal areas accentuated by increased numbers of chronic inflammatory cells, including monocytes, lymphocytes, and plasma cells. There is significant interface hepatitis with portal–central bridges and pseudorosette formation of periportal hepatocytes. There is also ballooning and acidophilic degeneration of liver cells (**128**).

ii. Autoimmune hepatitis is caused by cytotoxic lymphocytes infiltrating the liver in an HLA susceptible patient, as a consequence of disordered immunoregulation. A defect in suppressor T cell regulation has been identified. The presence of certain MHC genes may promote disease susceptibility including class I and II antigens HLA A1, B8, DR3, and DR4. Each has been detected with increased frequency in patients with autoimmune hepatitis. MHC is involved in the process of (auto) antigen presentation and recognition, which may initiate cellular and humoral responses against liver-specific proteins. Autoimmune hepatitis has a female preponderance (female to male ratio, 8:1). Half the patients present between 10 and 20 years old; a further peak of incidence is seen about the age of 50. The onset is usually insidious. However, in 25% of the cases, disease presents as a typical attack of acute viral hepatitis. The 10 year survival rates of untreated patients is <50%.

iii. Autoimmune hepatitis is associated with ulcerative colitis, Hashimoto's thyroiditis, Coombs positive hemolytic anemia, polyarthritis, and purpura have been described. Cushingoid appearance, acne, hirsutism, cutaneous striae, and amenorrhea may complicate autoimmune hepatitis type I in young women.

iv. Immunosuppressive treatment prolongs life in these patients. Prednisone or prednisolone is the mainstay of therapy, often used with azathioprine to allow maintenance treatment on a low dose of corticosteroids. Liver transplantation is effective in patients with end-stage disease.

129 i. B. The outlook is very good for a young woman and she has a better than 90% chance of surviving for more than 10 years. Although liver transplantation is only required in the minority of patients, the results are good and continuing to improve. A better than 70% 5 year survival rate can be anticipated.

ii. In the absence of cirrhosis, the risks associated with pregnancy are small and a normal outcome can be anticipated. If a pregnancy is planned, azathioprine can be withdrawn and prednisolone increased to compensate for the loss of steroid sparing effect of azathioprine. In any event the crucial point is to avoid relapse during pregnancy. (See also **147**.)

130 A 48-year-old male with alcoholic cirrhosis complains of tender breast enlargement. Current medications include multivitamins, cimetidine, thiamine, spironolactone, furosemide, and lactulose. Features of his examination are depicted (130a, b).

i. Comment on the illustrations.

ii. What other signs and symptoms are associated with this condition?

iii. What is the role of alcohol versus liver disease in this condition?

iv. How should this patient be treated?

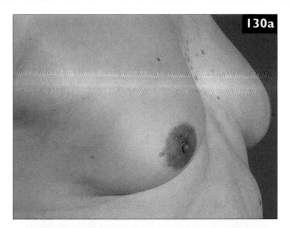

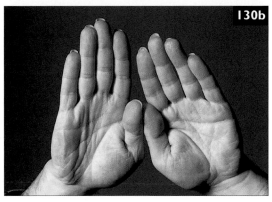

131 A 60-year-old, white male has moved to your area after retiring. He was diagnosed as having hemochromatosis 5 years previously. His liver biopsy at that time showed cirrhosis. He received aggressive phlebotomy therapy and has had complete depletion of his excess iron stores. He feels well except for occasional fatigue.

Albumin 3.2 g/dL (32 g/L)
Other liver chemistries normal
Prothrombin time slightly prolonged
Platelet count 110,000/mm³ (110 × 10⁹/L)
Fasting transferrin saturation 55%
Serum ferritin 58 ng/mL (1.04 µmol/L)

Laboratory investigations are shown. His last phlebotomy was four months ago.

i. What should you recommend for maintenance phlebotomy?

ii. Should this patient be screened for hepatocellular cancer? If so, how?

130 i. The illustrations depict gynecomastia (**130a**) and palmar erythema (**130b**).

ii. Sexual dysfunction with decreased libido and impotence, decreased facial, axillary and sternal hair, and testicular atrophy.

iii. Hypogonadism is common among men with chronic liver disease, but it is particularly frequent among those with alcoholic cirrhosis. In men with severe, nonalcoholic liver disease decreased testicular function is caused by dysregulation of hypothalamic–pituitary function related to the severity of the liver disease. In alcoholic patients, these changes are exacerbated by the direct effects of alcohol which produces testicular atrophy and decreases the production of testosterone by inhibiting the enzymes involved in its synthesis. In addition, ethanol increases both hepatic degradation of testosterone and the conversion of androgens to estrogens which contribute to feminization. Because of the direct gonadal toxicity, patients with alcoholic cirrhosis might have elevated gonadotropin levels in contrast to those with nonalcoholic liver disease in whom the levels are decreased.

iv. In alcoholic patients adverse drug reactions should always be considered. In men with nonalcoholic cirrhosis, spironolactone treatment is associated with gynecomastia and decreased testosterone levels with liver disease of intermediate severity. To prevent these side effects, the spironolactone should be discontinued. Instead, amiloride which is also effective in high aldosterone states but does not have this side effect should be used to treat this patient's fluid overload.

131 i. Maintenance phlebotomy of 1 unit of whole blood every 2–3 months is usually adequate. Once patients have been depleted of their excess iron stores with initial therapeutic phlebotomy, then maintenance phlebotomy is necessary usually for the rest of the patient's life. As patients with hereditary hemochromatosis usually absorb an increased amount of dietary iron in the order of 2–3 mg/day, they can absorb as much as 270 mg of iron over a 3 month period. Thus, phlebotomy of a single unit of whole blood containing approximately 250 mg of iron is usually sufficient to keep patients in normal iron balance. Occasional patients can require less frequent maintenance phlebotomy but transferrin saturation and ferritin levels should be monitored periodically. Transferrin saturation of <50% and ferritin <50 ng/mL (<3.95 µmol/L) are suggested goals.

ii. Screening for hepatocellular cancer in cirrhotic hemochromatosis is controversial. For those patients who desire screening or for those physicians who wish to do so, the recommendation is to obtain an ultrasound and alphafetoprotein level every 6–12 months. In patients with hemochromatosis, hepatocellular cancer was found at 200 times the frequency expected in an age- and gender-matched control population. Hepatocellular cancer rarely occurs in hemochromatosis patients without cirrhosis. Thus, screening for hepatocellular cancer is unnecessary in noncirrhotic patients once they have been successfully depleted of their excess iron stores. Hepatocellular cancer can develop in cirrhotic patients many years after excess iron stores have been depleted.

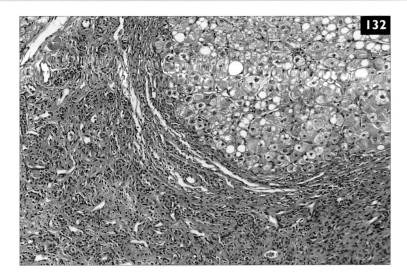

132 Percutaneous liver biopsy is often helpful in the evaluation of children with suspected liver disease. This biopsy was obtained and provided confirmation for a suspected diagnosis.

i. What is revealed in the liver biopsy (H&E) (**132**)?

ii. What therapy and management is suggested for children with tyrosinemia?

133 A 45-year-old cirrhotic patient with diagnosed ascites is admitted to the emergency room because of mid-abdominal pain of 3 days duration. On physical examination the patient is slightly febrile. Grade 2 hepatic encephalopathy, jaundice, and a distended and tender abdomen are noted. Laboratory investigations are shown.

i. Which is the most likely diagnosis?

ii. Should further diagnostic tests be ordered?

iii. Which treatment would you recommend?

Bilirubin 3 mg/dL (51.3 μmol/L)
WBC count 14,000/mm³ (14 × 10⁹/L)
Creatinine 2.8 mg/dL (247.5 μmol/L)
Platelet count 60,000/mm³ (60 × 10⁹/L)
BUN 56 mg/dL (urea 9.3 mmol/L)
Amylase 340 U/L
Ascitic fluid:
Protein 2.8 g/dL (28 g/L)
Polymorphonuclear leukocytes 4,000/mm³
 (4 × 10⁹/L)
LDH 800 U/L
Amylase 1,324 U/L
Glucose 43 mg/dL (2.39 mmol/L)
pH 7.35

132 i. This is a liver biopsy from a child with tyrosinemia. Note the micronodular cirrhosis, bile duct proliferation within portal tracts, and fibrotic septa. The hepatocytes have varying degrees of steatosis and appear in a 'pseudoglandular' arrangement around a central canaliculus. These findings are nonspecific and are frequently observed in a wide variety of neonatal liver disorders including neonatal hepatitis.

ii. Dietary restriction of phenylalanine, methionine, and of tyrosine are routinely advised. No large controlled study has been undertaken to confirm the long term beneficial effect of this regimen. Renal tubular abnormalities can be improved with dietary manipulation, but hepatic protection has not been documented. The risk of hepatocellular carcinoma in children with tyrosinemia demands systematic careful follow-up. As serum alphafetoprotein levels may already be elevated, alphafetoprotein can not serve as a useful marker for malignancy in these children. Ultrasound or CT examinations may be helpful for screening these children for nodules. The nature of hepatic nodules pose a clinical dilemma. Nodules may be hepatocellular carcinomas or regenerative nodules of cirrhosis. Any tyrosinemic child with nodules on CT scan or ultrasound should be considered for liver transplantation. Recently, much enthusiasm has surrounded the use of 2-(2-nitro-4-trifluoromethylbenzoyl)-cyclohexane-1,3-dione (NTBC) an inhibitor of 4-hydroxyphenylpyruvate dioxygenase, for the therapy of tyrosinemia. The drug has had some dramatic effects on neurologic crises, and has significantly improved hepatic and coagulation profiles. Unfortunately, in an animal model of tyrosinemia, NTBC has not prevented the development of hepatocellular carcinoma. Thus, currently NTBC should be used with caution in the long term with frequent surveillance for hepatocellular carcinoma development. Some texts recommend liver transplantation for all children with tyrosinemia before 2 years of age because of the great risk of hepatocellular carcinoma.

133 i. The ascitic fluid showed above fulfills two of the three criteria proposed to detect peritonitis associated with perforation (namely ascitic fluid total protein >1g/dL [>10 g/L], glucose <50 mg/dL [<2.8 mmol/L] and LDH greater than the upper limit of normality for serum). When two of these criteria are identified, sensitivity in detecting episodes of actual gut perforation is said to be 100% (although the specificity is low: 45%). In this case, both the severe systemic involvement and the symptomatology point to intestinal perforation as the most likely diagnosis. Note that a rigid abdomen does not usually develop in cirrhotics, even in cases of free perforation of viscera.

ii. Gastrografin enema, gastrointestinal series, and ultrasound examination are mandatory in order to rule out gut perforation. In this patient a gastrografin leak from the gastric antrum was noted.

iii. Laparotomy and surgical correction is the only available treatment. The mortality associated with such a procedure is exceedingly high.

134 What is the most effective treatment to decrease the risk of esophageal variceal hemorrhage? How should the dose of medication be determined and how would you best monitor the efficacy of treatment?

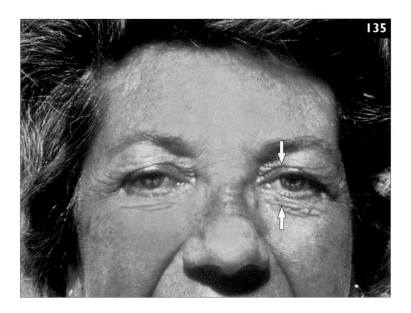

135 A 50-year-old female complains of mild itching. She is pigmented and abdominal examination reveals a 4 cm (1.6 in) enlarged liver and palpable spleen. Xanthalasmata were seen around both eyes (**135**).
i. What is the diagnosis?
ii. What tests should be performed to confirm the diagnosis?
iii. What treatment(s) should be considered?

134 Nonselective beta adrenergic blockers (propranolol and nadolol) provide the only effective means for reducing the risk of first variceal hemorrhage. Most trials determine the dose of nonselective beta adrenergic blockers by achieving a 25% reduction in resting heart rate, with the final heart rate of more than 55 beats/min. However, data from recent studies strongly support measurements of the hepatic venous pressure gradient at baseline and at 2–3 months with a goal of achieving a reduction of the hepatic venous pressure gradient of more than 20% and, or, a reduction to <12 mmHg (<1.6 kPa). There are seven published randomized controlled trials (five for propranolol, two for nadolol) and two studies published in abstract only comparing a nonselective beta adrenergic blocker to a placebo for the prevention of initial variceal bleeding. A meta-analysis of the studies shows an odds ratio of 0.52, 95% confidence interval, 0.30–0.71, (P<0.01). The studies are relatively homogenous and have received excellent scores for quality of design. Pooling data from these studies, beta adrenergic blockers achieve a 40% reduction in the risk of initial variceal hemorrhage. For patients achieving a reduction in the hepatic venous pressure gradient of more than 20% and, or, a reduction to <12 mmHg (<1.6 kPa), the risk of initial variceal bleeding is negligible. Based on the patient population included in these studies, the conclusions are applicable for patients with large esophageal varices and relatively good liver function. Very few patients with small esophageal varices or Child's class C cirrhosis were included in the studies. Subgroup analysis shows that patients classified as Child's B are most likely to benefit from beta blocker therapy. Recent studies have shown no benefit for patients treated with sclerotherapy for the prevention of initial variceal bleeding. Endoscopic banding, however, has shown more promising results in initial studies.

135 i. The most likely diagnosis is primary biliary cirrhosis. This is considered to be an autoimmune disease with a strong female predominance (female:male ratio 9:1).
ii. Serum biochemical tests show a cholestatic pattern with an elevated ALP and GGT. The specific diagnostic test is the antimitochondrial antibody test which is positive in over 90% of cases. Serum immunoglobulin levels show an elevated IgM concentration. An abdominal ultrasound should be performed to exclude extrahepatic obstruction. A liver biopsy should be carried out to confirm the diagnosis and determine the extent of liver damage.
iii. Symptomatic treatment consists of cholestyramine for itching. In view of the accelerated osteoporosis seen postmenopausally in this mainly female group of patients, treatment should be considered with either hormone replacement therapy or bisphosphonates. Fat soluble vitamin replacement is required in jaundiced patients.
Long term use of ursodeoxycholic acid in a dose of 10–15 mg/kg has been shown to reduce mortality and morbidity. Patients with advanced liver disease can be treated by liver transplantation with a 90–95% 5 year survival rate.

136 A 43-year-old African-American female was admitted to the hospital with nausea, vomiting, and fatigue of 5–7 days and jaundice of 2–3 days duration. Laboratory investigations are shown.

Her past medical history was only significant for a positive tuberculin skin test, for which she had been receiving oral isoniazid 600 mg daily for 2 months. Within 24 hours of admission, she develops lethargy and asterixis.

AST 1,640 U/L
ALT 1,872 U/L
Bilirubin 12.2 mg/dL (208.6 µmol/L)
Prothrombin time 26 seconds
HBsAg, IgM anti-HBc, and anti-HCV absent
Alpha-1-antitrypsin, ceruloplasmin, and ferritin levels normal
Antinuclear, smooth muscle and antimitochondrial antibodies absent

i. What is the most likely diagnosis?
ii. What would the liver biopsy most likely show?
iii. What is the pathogenesis of this clinical illness?
iv. What is the management of this clinical condition?

137 A newborn exhibits persistent jaundice, with a bilirubin of 22 mg/dL (376.2 µmol/L). A right upper quadrant ultrasound fails to image a gallbladder or bile ducts. Liver chemistries are otherwise normal.
i. Which of the following provides the most appropriate initial therapy:
A Phototherapy.
B Kasai portoenterostomy (**137**).
C Liver transplantation.
D Parenteral nutrition.
ii. What are other indications for liver transplantation in children?

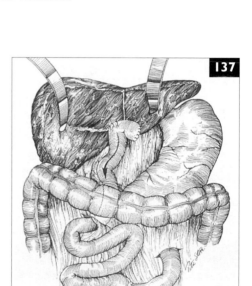

136 i. Isoniazid induced hepatitis. The clinical features are indistinguishable from viral hepatitis, with patients often complaining of malaise, anorexia, and nausea before jaundice develops. Biochemically, it also mimics viral hepatitis-like illness with jaundice as a presenting feature in 10% of patients. Individuals over the age of 40 are more likely to develop hepatotoxicity, with fatality higher in African–American women. Almost half of affected patients develop symptoms within 2 months of initiation of treatment; the remainder present as late as 11 months after treatment is begun.
ii. Liver biopsy in patients with established hepatitis reveals diffuse hepatocellular necrosis. In fatal cases, massive necrosis may be found. In a few patients, there have been features on liver biopsy of chronic hepatitis and cirrhosis.
iii. Isoniazid induced hepatic necrosis is probably the result of production of toxic intermediate metabolites of the drug, which are highly reactive moieties that can bind covalently to cell macromolecules and lead to cell necrosis. Production of toxic intermediates appears to explain the mildly elevated aminotransferase levels with minimal hepatic necrosis observed early in the course of treatment in 10–20% of patients and which resolves completely in the vast majority despite continued treatment. Formation of toxic intermediates may also explain the 1% incidence of severe necrosis.
iv. Treatment is entirely supportive, as for acute viral hepatitis. Corticosteroids are of no established value. Prevention or early detection of significant isoniazid induced hepatitis has proved elusive.

137 i. B. Kasai portoenterostomy. This patient exhibits the classic presentation of extrahepatic biliary atresia. This condition is a developmental failure of the entire bile ductular system and leads to persistent jaundice and biliary cirrhosis if not treated promptly. There is no role for phototherapy in this disorder, because the liver conjugates bilirubin normally, and the problem is one of obstruction. Parenteral nutrition likewise will have no effect on outcome. The two options for treatment are portoenterostomy and liver transplantation. The Kasai procedure accomplishes drainage of vestigial bile ductular structures into a Roux-en-Y limb of small intestine. One third of patients can be expected to obtain long term relief with this procedure. One third achieve short term relief but ultimately require transplantation. If these patients thrive and grow in the interim, the chances of success with liver transplantation later are significantly increased. One third of patients have no bile ductule and require a transplant. Ninety per cent of patients who do not receive successful drainage with the procedure and who do not undergo transplantation die within 5 years. Persistent attempts at reoperation for failure of a Kasai procedure have been shown to worsen the outcome of liver transplantation. Most centers advocate an initial Kasai portoenterostomy followed by liver transplantation immediately in patients in whom the procedure fails or at the time of recurrent jaundice.
ii. Extrahepatic biliary atresia occurs in 1 of 15,000 live births and accounts for 50–60% of pediatric transplants. It is more common in males. Alagille's syndrome, or arteriohepatic dysplasia, is the next most common indication, followed by metabolic deficiencies such as alpha-1-antitrypsin deficiency and Wilson's disease. Another common pediatric indication is fulminant hepatic failure of unknown etiology.

138 A 34-year-old male presents with bleeding esophageal varices and is found on examination to have hepatosplenomegaly and mild jaundice. His hepatic synthetic function is normal. An ultrasound scan confirms hepatosplenomegaly and multiple cysts within the liver associated with a dilated common bile duct.

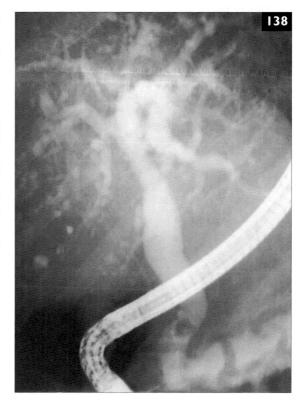

i. What two abnormalities are shown in this ERCP (138)?
ii. What medical conditions occur in this disease?
iii. What is the prognosis?

139 A 54-year-old, white male is referred for further evaluation of an elevated transferrin saturation accompanied by an increased ferritin level. He complains of fatigue, arthralgias, and impotence. His physical examination shows skin pigmen-

ALT 85 U/L
AST 60 U/L
Serum albumin 3.3 g/dL (33 g/L)
Total bilirubin normal
ALP normal
Serum ferritin 1,825 ng/mL (32.67 µmol/L)
Transferrin saturation 98%

tation, hepatomegaly, and arthritic changes in the hands. Laboratory investigations are shown. A percutaneous liver biopsy is performed which shows 4+ stainable iron predominantly in hepatocytes with early cirrhosis. Hepatic iron concentration is 28,270 µg/g with a calculated hepatic iron index of 9.3.
i. What is the likely diagnosis?
ii. How should this patient be treated?

138 i. Multiple sacular dilations of the intrahepatic biliary tree and mild dilation of the extrahepatic biliary tree. The second abnormality is a gallstone in the lower part of the common bile duct. The principal diagnosis is Caroli's syndrome. This is an inherited biliary condition characterised by sacular diverticula in the hepatic bile ducts. The abnormality may be restricted to one part of the liver, or as in this case, be found throughout. The diverticula are predisposed to infection and stone formation.

ii. Caroli's syndrome is strongly associated with congenital hepatic fibrosis. In this patient bleeding varices were a consequence of portal hypertension caused by congenital hepatic fibrosis rather than a direct consequence of the Caroli's syndrome. A second association is medullary sponge kidney.

iii. The outcome in this patient relates to the management of portal hypertension. Patients who have portal hypertension resulting from congenital hepatic fibrosis have excellent hepatic synthetic function and are strong candidates for portacaval shunt or TIPS. The prognosis of the biliary disease is uncertain. Caroli's syndrome is associated with a malignant transformation of the biliary tree on a background of recurrent cholangititis and stone formation and are at risk from consequent hepatic damage. Treatment is, therefore, based upon alleviation of biliary sepsis. Biliary sphincterotomy and frequent use of antibiotics are necessary for patients who develop stones. Liver transplantation may be necessary.

139 i. Idiopathic hemochromatosis.

ii. The patient should be treated with weekly phlebotomy. This patient presents with classic hereditary hemochromatosis but unfortunately was diagnosed after the development of cirrhosis and fairly significant symptoms. One study has shown a 'hepatic iron concentration threshold' for the development of fibrosis and, or, cirrhosis in otherwise uncomplicated patients of approximately 22,000 µg/g; this patient is above that threshold. Treatment should be with weekly phlebotomy of 1 unit (500 mL) of whole blood. This

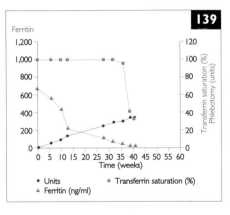

is equivalent to approximately 250 mg of iron. If patients can tolerate 1 unit of blood two times per week, that can be suggested. It is anticipated that with the degree of iron-loading seen in this patient, up to 1 year or more of weekly phlebotomy will be necessary to deplete the excess iron stores. Typically, the serum ferritin gradually decreases with the gradual reduction of total body iron stores but the transferrin saturation will remain elevated until just before the excess iron stores are depleted (**139**). It is reasonable to obtain iron studies every 3 months or so to monitor the reduction in ferritin in order to predict return to normal iron stores with serum ferritin <50 ng/mL.

140 A 44-year-old male teacher diagnosed with ulcerative colitis 8 years previously has had fluctuating biochemical liver test results with temporarily increased levels of both aminotransferase and ALP levels for 5 years. Hepatitis B and C tests were negative. An ERCP undertaken 3 years ago showed normal bile ducts. The patient has no abdominal pain but occasional spells of pruritus. The colitis was brought into remission for several years with the aid of sulfasalazine (two 500 mg tablets twice a day).

The patient was not consuming excess alcohol. There were no signs of liver disease and no hepato- or splenomegaly. He is anxious regarding the cause of his abnormal liver tests.

What further investigations should be done to give him a proper answer?

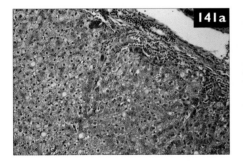 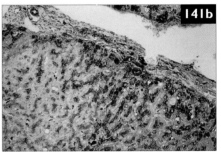

141 A 48-year-old male was initially evaluated for arthritic symptoms involving multiple joints, but was found to have abnormal biochemical liver test results shown. A subsequent laboratory screen for viral, immunologic, and genetic etiologies of liver disease was negative. The patient underwent liver biopsy.

AST 70 U/L
ALT 86 U/L
Transferrin saturation 86%
Serum ferritin 1,840 ng/mL

i. Describe the biopsy findings (**141a**).
ii. Describe the biopsy findings (**141b**).
iii. Quantitative iron on liver biopsy was 18,640 µg/g dry weight. Calculate the hepatic iron index.
iv. How rapidly can iron be removed by phlebotomy therapy?
v. What are the results of liver transplantation for hemochromatosis?

140 A liver biopsy should be performed. The liver test results and the history of ulcerative colitis in this patient raises the suspicion of primary sclerosing cholangitis, but as his ERCP was normal he does not fulfill the criteria for this ailment. Other causes of abnormal liver tests have to be looked for. Treatment with sulfasalazine can lead to abnormal biochemical liver tests, but this patient had stopped taking medication without any effect on these test results. Chronic viral hepatitis and over consumption of alcohol do not usually cause cholestasis and were ruled out in this patient. No mitochondrial autoantibodies, smooth muscle antibodies, or antinuclear antibodies have been found. However, the patient was found to have antineutrophil antibodies. Almost 80% of all the patients with ulcerative colitis with or without primary sclerosing cholangitis have antineutrophil antibodies. The antineutrophil antibodies seen in patients with ulcerative colitis and primary sclerosing cholangitis differ from those seen in vasculitic disorders. Antineutrophil antibodies in vasculitic disorders have a diffuse cytoplasmic pattern (C-ANCA). In ulcerative colitis and primary sclerosing cholangitis the distribution is perinuclear (P-ANCA). It is unlikely that P-ANCA contributes to the pathogenesis of ulcerative colitis or primary sclerosing cholangitis but is a marker for an immunological disturbance in these patients. A repeat ERCP was performed, still showing normal bile ducts. However, in the liver biopsy, changes compatible with primary sclerosing cholangitis were seen. This patient can, therefore, be included in a small group of primary sclerosing cholangitis patients only having involvement of the small bile ducts. This is known as 'small bile duct sclerosing cholangitis'.

141 i. The most prominent finding on this biopsy is an amorphous brown pigmentation in the cytoplasm of hepatocytes.
ii. This biopsy is stained with an iron stain (Perls' Prussian blue stain) and demonstrates marked hepatocyte iron deposition.
iii. The hepatic iron index is calculated by dividing the hepatic iron content in mmol/g dry weight by the patient's age in years. Thus 18,640 divided by 56 (the molecular weight of iron, to convert mg to mmol) divided by 48 = 6.9. Values >2.0 are compatible with hereditary hemochromatosis.
iv. Phlebotomy typically is performed by removing 1 unit, or 500 mL, of blood on a weekly basis. One unit of blood contains 250 mg of iron. Thus, 1 g of iron will be removed in a month after four phlebotomies. As patients often have as much as 10–20 g of excess iron, phlebotomies may be required for 1–2 years.
v. Survival following liver transplantation for hemochromatosis has recently been reported to be significantly less than after transplantation performed for other conditions. In a recent institutional review and an analysis of Medicare data, the 1 year survival rate was approximately 55%, which is 25–30% less than the survival rate following liver transplantation for other liver diseases.

142 What is the Child's–Pugh score used for?

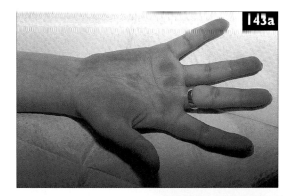

143 A 22-year-old female was seen because she had a 10 year history of relapsing ALT flares and increased serum IgG. Initially, she developed fatigue, dark urine, and jaundice over a 2 month period. She tested negative for HBsAg, antibody to smooth muscle, nuclear and mitochondrial antigens. She denied alcohol, parenteral drug abuse, and exposure to the risk factors for viral hepatitis. Liver biopsy showed mild lymphocytic portal infiltration and she was left untreated. Her present physical examination shows jaundice, hepato-splenomegaly, and several spider angio-mata. Laboratory investigations are shown. Abdominal ultrasound shows enlargement of liver and spleen with focal lesions. A liver biopsy was performed. An upper gastrointestinal endoscopy was carried out.
i. Comment on figure 143a.
ii. Comment on the upper gastrointestinal endoscopy findings (143b).

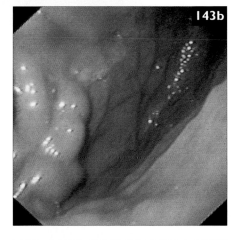

ALT 391 U/L
AST 280 U/L
Bilirubin 5.9 mg/dL (100.9 mmol/L)
Albumin 4.0 g/dL (40 g/L)
Gammaglobulin 2.8 g/dL (28 g/L)
Anti-HCV absent
Smooth muscle antibodies absent
Antinuclear antibodies absent
Antimitochondrial antibodies absent
Anti-liver-kidney microsomal antibodies 1: 320

Criterion		Score
Encephalopathy	None	1
	Easy to control	
	Precipitating cause	2
	Recurrent. No cause	
	Difficult to control	3
Ascites	Absent	1
	Easy to control. Slight	2
	Diuretic resistant	
	Moderate-tense	3
Bilirubin mg/dL (µmol/L)	<2 (<34.2)	1
	2–3 (34.2–51.3)	2
	>3 (>51.3)	3
Albumin g/dL (g/L)	>3.5 (>35)	1
	2.8–3.5 (28–35)	2
	<2.8 (<28)	3
Prothrombin time	1–4	1
(seconds prolonged)	4–6	2
	>6	2

Child's–Pugh classification: a total score 5–6, B total score 7–9, C total score 10–15.

142 The Child's–Pugh classification is in wide use as the measure of severity of chronic liver disease. The classification has high predictive value for survival in patients with cirrhosis. The Child's–Pugh classification uses a point scoring system, assigned by assessing physical findings and laboratory data. The total points determine the assignment of a classification A, B, or C according to the criteria shown in the above table.

143 i. **143a** shows palmar erythema, i.e. exaggerated red flushing of the palms affecting the thenar and hypothenar eminences and the bases of the fingers. It is seen in liver disease, pregnancy, thyrotoxicosis, and bronchial carcinoma. It may also be a genetically determined characteristic.
ii. Fiberoptic endoscopy is employed to detect esophageal varices. This endoscopic picture of the lower end of the esophagus (**143b**) shows large submucosal varices. Large submucosal varices in the esophagus can also be demonstrated radiologically by a barium swallow examination. Esophageal varices are classified by size. The presence of red signs on varices, as well as large size, are predictors of future bleeding.

144 With regard to **143**:
i. Comment on the recently taken liver biopsy (**144a, b**).
ii. What is the diagnosis of this condition?
iii. How many types of liver-kidney microsomal antibodies exist?
iv. What is the natural history of this condition?
v. What treatment is indicated for this patient?

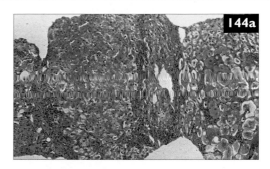

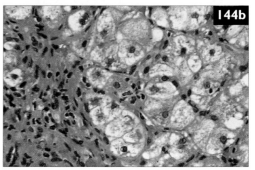

145 A 43-year-old alcoholic female presents with a 1 month history of watery diarrhea, abdominal discomfort, anorexia, and significant weight loss. The patient was diagnosed with alcoholic liver cirrhosis 3 years before, but no decompensation had occurred. She denied fever or any other symptomatology. On physical examination a poor nutritional status, chronic liver disease stigmata, and ascites were detected, with no other abnormalities. A paracentesis was performed and the laboratory results and remaining investigations are shown.
i. What is revealed by the ascitic fluid analysis?
ii. Could any other laboratory investigation be useful?
iii. Which would be the definite diagnostic procedure?

Paracentesis results:
Total protein 3.9 g/dL (39 g/L)
Albumin 1.5 g/dL (15 g/L)
LDH 359 U/L
Glucose 98 mg/dL (5.44 mmol/L)
Nucleated cells 1,300/mm³
   (95% mononuclear)
Triglycerides 80 mg/dL (0.9 mmol/L)
Ascitic fluid negative Ziehl–Neelsen stain
No atypical cells in ascitic fluid

Other investigations:
WBC count 4,100/mm³ (4.1 × 10⁹/L)
Platelet count 120,000/mm³ (120 × 10⁹/L)
Gammaglobulin 1.8 g/dL (18 g/L)
Bilirubin 2 mg/dL (34.2 μmol/L)
Plasma albumin 2.7 g/dL (27 g/L)
ESR 5 mm (first hour)
HIV serology negative

144 i. The liver biopsy shows nodular transformation of the hepatic parenchyma indicating cirrhosis has developed. There is interface hepatitis and areas of collapse containing trapped hepatocytes (**144a**). There is Mallory hyalin in liver cells of the lobular periphery with pigment indicating peripheral cholestasis. Mallory's hyalin in the liver cells of central areas would suggest alcoholic liver disease. A distinctive feature of autoimmune hepatitis is the 'pseudorosette' formation at the periphery of portal tracts, i.e. hepatocytes showing a pseudoductular arrangement surrounded by inflammatory cells.

ii. This patient has autoimmune hepatitis type II leading to cirrhosis and portal hypertension.

iii. There are three types of liver-kidney microsomal antibodies (anti-LKM) These antibodies appear in true autoimmune hepatitis (anti-LKM_1), drug induced hepatitis (anti-LKM_2) and hepatitis D (anti-LKM_3). The molecular target of anti-LKM_1, anti-LKM_2, and anti-LKM_3 are cytochromes P450 2D6, 2C9, and 1A2, respectively.

iv. Typical patients with autoimmune hepatitis type II are young, 90% female with elevated inflammatory hepatic indices. An association with HLA-DR3 and C4A-Q0 has been described. If untreated, disease progresses to cirrhosis in a few years.

v. Immunosuppression may be very effective therapy. In most patients however, treatment with steroids with or without azathioprine may not prevent development of cirrhosis. Liver transplantation is effective in patients with end-stage disease.

145 i. The ascitic fluid exhibits a high protein concentration but with a serum-ascites albumin gradient >1.1 g/dL (11 g/L), which points to portal hypertension as the most probable cause of the ascites. However, the presence of an increased number of ascitic lymphocytes and the high ascitic LDH level suggest that other conditions may contribute, especially lymphoma, ovarian tumors, peritoneal carcinomatosis, or tuberculous peritonitis. The absence of atypical cells argues against ovarian or peritoneal carcinomatosis. Lymphoma is characterized by a high triglyceride ascitic fluid concentration (chylous ascites). Alcoholism and, or, liver cirrhosis are well known risk factors for tuberculous peritonitis, which in this setting usually present insidiously, without fever, with a negative tuberculin skin test, and in the absence of remarkable ascitic fluid abnormalities.

ii. A Ziehl–Neelsen stain of ascitic fluid is often negative. Although Lowenstein cultures are very sensitive, they take several weeks to become positive. The assessment of the adenosine deaminase value in ascitic fluid (diagnostic when >35 U/L) is a parameter with great sensitivity and specificity and very useful in this setting.

iii. The diagnosis of tuberculous peritonitis should be definitively proved through a laparoscopic peritoneal biopsy.

146 A 52-year-old male is referred for the evaluation of abnormal liver tests. He admits to drinking half a pint of bourbon daily. Review of symptoms is remarkable for impotence for the previous 2 years. Physical examination reveals spider angiomata, gynecomastia, hepatosplenomegaly, and testicular atrophy.

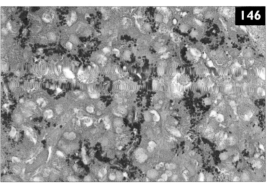

Laboratory investigations are shown. Percutaneous liver biopsy is illustrated (146, courtesy of Dr Maria Leo-Lieber).

i. What is the differential diagnosis of the patient's cirrhosis based on the non-invasive tests?
ii. Comment on the liver biopsy findings.
iii. What is the role of iron in alcoholic liver disease?
iv. What is the differential diagnosis of the hypogonadism in alcoholic patients with liver disease and possible iron overload?
v. What physical findings suggest the cause of this patient's hypogonadism?
vi. Interpret the endocrine test results.
vii. What tests are available to determine the role of elevated serum iron levels in alcoholic patients with liver disease?

Hemoglobin 14.2 g/dL (142 g/L)
MCV 102.4 fL (mm³)
Prothrombin time 14.8 seconds
AST 80 U/L
ALT 28 U/L
Albumin 3.2 g/dL (32 g/L)
Total bilirubin 1.8 mg/dL (30.8 mol/L)
ALP 112 U/L
GGTP 200 U/L
Iron 180 µg/dL (32.2 µmol/L)
TIBC 200 µg/dL (35.8 µmol/L)
Ferritin 800 ng/mL
Testosterone 88 ng/dL
Estrogen 111 ng/dL
Luteinizing hormone 12.2 U/L
HBAg absent
Anti-HCV absent

147 The patient in 129 with autoimmune hepatitis is now on azathioprine 50 mg/day and prednisolone 10 mg/day. Biochemical liver tests have been normal for 2 years but she now complains of weight gain, acne, and a change in her facial features which you consider typically 'Cushingoid'. Her mother thinks the patient is missing some doses of prednisolone because she blames the drug for her changing features. What do you advise?
A A trial withdrawal of all treatment as in most instances steroids can be withdrawn.
B Gradually reducing corticosteroids until the side effects disappear.
C Offer a higher dose of azathioprine and withdrawal of the prednisolone.
D Advise that she should continue current treatment indefinitely.

146 i. Alcoholic liver disease with iron overload versus genetic hemochromatosis are the main considerations in the differential diagnosis.

ii. The liver biopsy reveals iron overload which is predominantly located in reticuloendothelial cells. In genetic hemochromatosis, abundant iron is present mainly within hepatocytes. Iron in biliary cells may also occasionally be seen.

iii. In early studies of hemochromatosis, the role of iron as an hepatotoxin was questioned as many of the affected patients were also alcoholic. Ethanol facilitates iron absorption and can potentially exacerbate this hereditary condition. Conversely, iron also potentiates experimental ethanol toxicity by increasing lipid peroxidation.

iv. Men with nonalcoholic cirrhosis frequently have evidence of hypogonadism which correlates with the degree of hepatic impairment. Patients with alcoholic cirrhosis and genetic hemochromatosis, however, are more severely afflicted. Primary testicular failure can result from direct alcohol toxicity. In genetic hemochromatosis, secondary hypogonadism develops as a result of iron overload of the anterior pituitary.

v. Impotence as a manifestation of hypoandrogenism is frequent in both alcoholic cirrhosis and genetic hemochromatosis. Clinical evidence of hyperestrogenism (gynecomastia and palmar erythema) and elevated estrogen levels are very common in alcoholics but rare in patients with genetic hemochromatosis.

vi. In patients with alcoholic cirrhosis, reduced levels of plasma testosterone are associated with increased levels of luteinizing hormone. In genetic hemochromatosis, levels of both testosterone and luteinizing hormone (due to anterior pituitary involvement) are low. Estrogenic activity is normal in patients with hemochromatosis. However, there is increased conversion of androgens to estrogens in alcoholic cirrhosis. As a result, estradiol and estrone levels are normal in the former and elevated in the latter condition.

vii. Liver biopsy with iron quantification and calculation of the hepatic iron index to adjust for patient age and, or, response to phlebotomy therapy once were the means to distinguish genetic hemochromatosis from alcoholic liver disease with iron overload. However, genetic testing for genetic hemochromatosis is now available.

147 C. If the azathioprine dose is increased to 2 mg/kg bodyweight then in 70% of cases steroids can be completely withdrawn with the abolition of steroid side-effects. If the initial diagnosis is confident, the likelihood of being able to withdraw all treatment is small and potentially dangerous. Likewise reducing the dose of steroids without increasing the azathioprine dose is likely to lead to relapse. If either of these courses is employed weekly surveillance of biochemical liver tests is mandatory for early diagnosis of relapse. Although continuing current treatment indefinitely may be theoretically appropriate for good survival it is likely that the patient will stop treatment and undergo relapse.

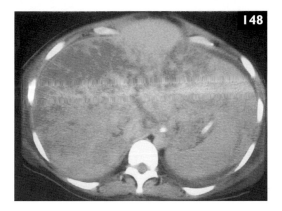

148 A 31-year-old Caucasian female who is 39 weeks pregnant presents with right upper abdominal pain, nausea, vomiting, headache, and recent obvious weight gain. Examination reveals an ill looking pale woman with a pulse rate of 120 beats/min, blood pressure 140/110 mmHg (18.7/14.7 kPa), no jaundice but marked peripheral edema, and a tender gravid abdomen. Urine testing was highly protein positive. Laboratory investigations are shown. An urgent CT scan was performed (148).

Hemoglobin 7.5 g/dL (75 g/L)
WBC count 20,000/mm³ (20 × 10⁹/L)
Platelet count 70,000/mm³ (70 × 10⁹/L)
Bilirubin 2.9 mg/dL (49.6 µmol/L)
AST 4,000 U/L
LDH 3,000 U/L
ALP 590 U/L
GGT 40 U/L
Albumin 3 g/dL (30 g/L)
Prothrombin time 24 seconds
Creatinine 2.03 mg/dL (0.18 mmol/L)
Potassium 4.5 mEq/L (4.5 mmol/L)
BUN 33 mg/dL (urea 5.5 mmol/L)

i. What is your provisional diagnosis?
ii. What does the CT scan show?
iii. What is the best management strategy and why?

149 A 6-year-old female begins having forceful vomiting and retching 3 days following the onset of varicella. Over the course of the next day she develops an alteration in consciousness and progresses through obtundation, delirium, and finally deep coma with tachypnea and extensor posturing. Physical examination reveals the child is anicteric with hepatomegaly. Laboratory investigations are shown.

Total bilirubin 1.2 mg/dL (20.5 µmol/L)
ALT 1,200 U/L
AST 1,125 U/L
Plasma ammonia 204 µg/dL (120 µmol/L)
Prothrombin time 16 seconds

What is the likely diagnosis?

153

148 i. Proteinuria, diastolic hypertension, and edema indicate pre-eclampsia. The triad of hemolysis, elevated liver enzymes, and low platelets constitutes HELLP syndrome. It can complicate up to 10% of cases of severe eclampsia. It is characterized by marked coagulopathy and platelet infarction of many organs particularly the brain, liver, and kidneys. The large elevation in AST and LDH in this setting suggests hepatic infarction. The differential diagnosis includes thrombotic thrombocytopenic purpura, hemolytic uremic syndrome, complicated cirrhosis, and fulminant hepatic failure from other causes.

ii. The CT scan accurately identifies hepatic infarction, a life threatening complication of HELLP. The multiple infarcts shown on this CT, were responsible for the high aminotransferase activities in this case. Ultrasound scan and Doppler flow studies will exclude thrombosis, e.g. in hepatic veins. MRI can also show hepatic infarction and vein clots.

iii. Resuscitation should correct any fluid deficits optimizing renal perfusion and coagulopathy should be reversed to minimize postpartum bleeding. Urgent delivery is essential to arrest the HELLP process. Perinatal infant mortality can approach 35%. There is also a high maternal death rate, usually from hepatic rupture complicating extensive hepatic infarction. Pre-eclampsia affects up to 10% of pregnancies, more so in first or multiple gestation pregnancies (e.g. twins) but is only severe in a minority of these. As with pre-eclampsia there is no increased risk of recurrence of the condition in later pregnancies.

149 The likely diagnosis for this child is Reye's syndrome. This syndrome is characterized by encephalopathy, liver dysfunction, and fatty infiltration of the viscera. The etiology of Reye's syndrome is unknown. However, it is often associated with a prodromal influenza or varicella infection. Abnormalities in urea cycle enzymes may be involved in the pathogenesis of this disorder. The essential diagnostic criteria for Reye's syndrome are the acute onset of a noninflammatory encephalopathy, elevated AST and ALT, a normal or near normal total bilirubin level, and fatty change on histologic review of the liver. Supportive of the diagnosis are hypoglycemia especially in small children, a prolonged prothrombin time, and elevated plasma ammonia level. The use of aspirin antecedent to Reye's syndrome was a statistically and clinically significant risk factor for developing Reye's syndrome. In 1982, the US Surgeon General issued an advisory cautioning the use of aspirin in children with influenza or varicella. No such correlation was found when examining the use of acetaminophen as an antipyretic in children with similar illness. Pediatricians and parents abandoned the use of aspirin for children with fever and the incidence of Reye's syndrome dropped significantly. In 1986 a mandatory warning about Reye's syndrome and aspirin use was placed on aspirin labels.

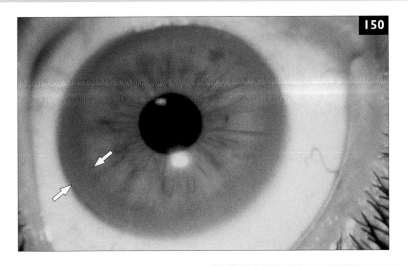

150 A 54-year-old female who was diagnosed as having Wilson's disease 20 years ago was seen for a follow-up examination. Her neurologic and hepatic signs and symptoms had abated with penicillamine. Family members say she seems somewhat distracted and agitated, and her handwriting has become progressively illegible and smaller in size. Clinical examination shows no change in the mild splenomegaly but mild dysarthria and tremors were noted. Laboratory investigations are shown. Slit-lamp examination was positive for Kayser–Fleischer rings (150, arrows).

Hemoglobin 12 g/dL (120 g/L)
Platelet count 100,000/mm³ (100 × 10⁹/L)
ALT 105 U/L
AST 80 U/L
ALP 100 U/L
Albumin 2.8 g/dL (28 g/L)
Ceruloplasmin 5 mg/dL (50 mg/L)
Serum copper 400 µg/L (6.3 µmol/L)
Urine copper 100 µg/24 hours
   (1.57 µmol/24 hours)

i. What is the most likely cause for her neurologic symptoms and signs of active liver disease?
ii. What testing or treatment should be performed?

151 Patients with chronic alcoholism and alcoholic hepatitis may present with abnormal mental status. Recognizing the possible presence of decompensated liver disease or alcohol withdrawal, how should these patients be treated?

150 i. The likely cause for her recurrent symptoms is noncompliance with treatment for Wilson's disease. This noncompliance is seen as recurrence of neurologic symptoms, behavioral changes, biochemical evidence of liver disease, and abnormalities of copper metabolism. This includes the recurrence of Kayser–Fleischer rings which should have disappeared during her first year of treatment and not recurred. Another parameter indicative of noncompliance is the elevated nonceruloplasmin bound copper. This value, normally <100 µg/L in treated patients, is approximately 350 µg/L in this patient. This value is derived from the difference of the total serum copper and the estimated amount of copper in ceruloplasmin, which is 0.3% of the weight of the protein. The final parameter of noncompliance is the urinary copper excretion of only 100 µg/24 hours. In patients treated with penicillamine, this value exceeds 1 g in the initial phases of treatment and is usually more than 500 µg/day in treated patients. While the 100 µg in this patient is above the normal range of copper excretion, it would have been higher if the patient had been taking the prescribed penicillamine.
ii. The reinitiation of penicillamine treatment is all that is necessary. Often patients who have discontinued their medications may deny doing so, and obtaining a simultaneous serum copper and ceruloplasmin, urinary copper excretion, and a slit-lamp examination as performed in this patient would indicate noncompliance before significant neurologic or hepatic disease has occurred. A simple but often neglected means of detection is also a pill count or check with the pharmacist to see if prescriptions for medication have been renewed. The failure to reinitiate appropriate therapy can result in further progression to crippling neurologic disease and to liver failure.

151 Thiamine should be administered to all patients, and hypoglycemia (after thiamine) and electrolyte disturbances (especially hypokalemia and hypophosphatemia) treated. If hepatic encephalopathy is present, precipitants (infection such as spontaneous bacterial peritonitis, upper gastrointestinal bleeding, prerenal azotemia, and hypokalemia) should be sought and treated, and the patient given lactulose. In encephalopathic patients with superimposed severe alcoholic hepatitis who do not have systemic infection or gastrointestinal bleeding, steroid therapy improves survival. Patients with symptoms of alcohol withdrawal should be treated with benzodiazepines because severe withdrawal resulting in delirium tremens carries a 15% mortality rate. However, a 'standing detox schedule' should not be written but rather the patient should be closely monitored and given doses as needed. All benzodiazepines are probably equally effective in treating alcohol withdrawal. It has been suggested that short-acting agents such as alprazolam, lorazepam, or oxazepam be used rather than longer-acting ones such as chlordiazepoxide which require hepatic metabolism. However, caution should be exercised with lorazepam as fatal respiratory arrest has been reported with its parenteral use in acutely intoxicated patients. Finally, ethanol appears to have a direct neurotoxic effect that contributes to chronic cognitive dysfunction in alcoholics, particularly those with liver disease or thiamine deficiency. There is a 'reversible' organic brain syndrome in chronic alcoholics that improves with 1 week of abstinence.

152 A 40-year-old male was admitted to hospital for evaluation of the recent onset of jaundice. He also complains of nausea, vague epigastric, and right upper quadrant discomfort but no severe pain. The patient estimates his daily alcohol intake to be 1 pint of vodka. He asserts that he has never used intravenous drugs, been transfused, or had homosexual contact. Recently he had an upper respiratory illness and difficulty in sleeping for which he used, over several days, a number of over-the-counter preparations containing variable amounts of acetaminophen (paracetamol) before hospital admission. On physical examination, he was alert and orientated, and clearly jaundiced. There were no cutaneous or other signs suggestive of liver disease. The heart and lungs were normal, but there was tenderness in the right upper quadrant, but no hepatomegaly. Laboratory investigations are shown. A transjugular liver biopsy was performed (152).

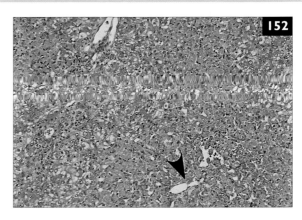

AST 14,800 U/L
ALT 6,720 U/L
Bilirubin 11.2 mg/dL (191.5 µmol/L)
ALP 70 U/L
Albumin 4.6 g/dL (46 g/L)
Prothrombin time 21 seconds
Creatinine 1.4 mg/dL (124 µmol/L)
WBC count 6,900/mm³ (6.9 × 10⁹/L)

i. Comment on the liver histology, in particular the area indicated by the arrow (152).
ii. What is the most likely diagnosis?
iii. What is the pathogenesis of this clinical illness?
iv. What is the management of this condition?

153 A 42-year-old male presents with a history of having had an abdominal ultrasound examination for a suspected kidney stone. The examination revealed an irregular mass in the anterior aspect of the liver. Biochemical liver tests were normal and the patient was asymptomatic. The patient had no history of liver disease and serum alphafetoprotein was normal.
i. What is the most common hepatic lesion to present in this manner?
ii. What imaging studies may confirm your diagnosis?

152 i. The liver histology shows centrilobular necrosis. Note the prominent eosinophilic change displayed by dead centrilobular hepatocytes (arrow). Periportal (zone 1) hepatocytes are spared but show swelling.

ii. Inadvertent acetaminophen (paracetamol) hepatotoxicity in an alcoholic patient.

iii. When taken in therapeutic doses, acetaminophen is predominantly eliminated via hepatic conjugation with sulfate and glucuronic acids. Approximately 5% of ingested acetaminophen is metabolized by the mixed function oxidase enzymes, primarily cytochrome P450 2E1. The main product of P450 2E1 oxidation is N-acetyl-p-benzo-quinoneimine (NAPQI), a highly reactive compound that is responsible for the toxic effects of acetaminophen. The small amount of NAPQI formed with therapeutic doses of acetaminophen is readily rendered nontoxic by conjugation with the intracellular tripeptide glutathione. Hepatotoxicity usually occurs with large doses of acetaminophen (>15 g in adults). This amount exceeds the capacity of the glucuronidation and sulfation pathways and results in the generation of large amounts of NAPQI. As a result of this, glutathione is rapidly consumed and hepatic stores depleted. Free NAPQI then reacts with (arylates) hepatic macromolecules, leading to the formation of covalent adducts with subsequent alteration in protein and hence cellular function. The mechanisms responsible for the development of hepatic necrosis with doses of acetaminophen within the therapeutic range in chronic alcohol users include induction of P450 2EI expression by alcohol, resulting in increased rates of production of NAPQI, and also depletion of hepatic glutathione by alcohol.

iv. The goals of management are threefold: reduce further absorption of the ingested acetaminophen; replete hepatic glutathione through administration of N-acetyl-cysteine; and institute supportive care for established hepatic failure. The mainstay of therapy is the administration of N-acetylcysteine, which promotes glutathione synthesis in the liver.

153 i. Cavernous hemangiomas are commonly present in this way.

ii. CT scanning with dynamic bolus intravenous contrast of hemangiomas may show characteristic contrast enhancement filling in from the periphery of the tumor, with persistent pooling of contrast on delayed films. No persistence of contrast is seen with hepatocellular adenomas. Focal nodular hyperplasia has

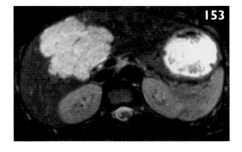

a classical appearance on CT scan of a central 'stellate' scar from fibrosis of the tumor. Sulfur colloid liver scans are not helpful. 99mTc-tagged red cell scan, especially if performed with single photon emission CT, is useful in the diagnosis of hemangioma. MRI can provide additional information; T1 images are usually hypointense in hepatocellular carcinoma and cysts, but iso- or hyperintense in the presence of fat and glycogen in hepatocellular adenomas. MRI is very sensitive in its ability to detect hemangiomas. The T2 weighted images give high signal intensity (**153**).

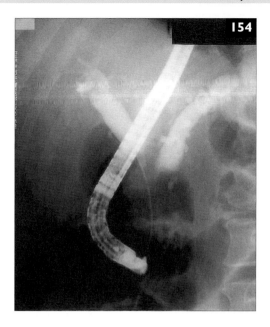

154 A 65-year-old female presents with obstructive jaundice and anemia. On examination she is found to have a palpable gallbladder. Fecal occult blood testing is strongly positive and her hemoglobin concentration is 7 g/dL (70 g/L). An endoscopy shows an ulcerated mass replacing the ampulla of Vater. Cholangiography and pancreatology are performed.
i. What abnormalities are seen on the ERCP (154)?
ii. Provide a likely description of the histological findings from biopsies of the duodenum.
iii. What further investigations should be considered?

155 A 43-year-old male tells you that he is to be screened for hemochromatosis as his 38-year-old brother was recently diagnosed with hemochromatosis by way of a liver biopsy. Your patient has no symptoms and a normal physical examination.
i. What blood studies should be performed?
ii. What is the value of HLA-typing and how reliable is the testing?

154 i. The ERCP shows dilation of both the common bile duct and the pancreas. This appearance is typical of ampullary cancer. The combination of anemia and obstructive jaundice strongly suggests this diagnosis. Periampullary tumors are often friable and bleed. Occasionally the combination of steatorrhea and gastrointestinal blood loss leads to the production of a silver colored stool.

ii. Histological examination would show well differentiated papillary adenocarcinoma. Ampullary carcinomas tend to occur in elderly subjects and are less common than pancreatic ductal tumors and cholangiocarcinoma.

iii. These tumors are often relatively slowly growing and have a relatively good prognosis with 25% survival at 5 years. Therefore, even in relatively elderly patients extensive staging procedures should be considered with a view to resectional surgery. Resection ideally comprises the Whipple's operation but local resection may also achieve good palliation. Final palliation by endoscopic laser treatment has also been described for inoperable tumors.

155 i. With the discovery of the hemochromatosis gene, HFE, screening has shifted to HFE mutation analysis. Whenever a diagnosis of hemochromatosis is made, it must be remembered that this is a hereditary disorder, inherited in an autosomal recessive fashion and that in addition to treating the patient, the primary physician has a responsibility to recommend family screening. Hereditary hemochromatosis is a common disorder affecting approximately 1 in 200 to 1 in 300 Caucasian individuals with a heterozygote frequency ranging between 1 in 8 to 1 in 12 individuals. In individuals <35 years of age, a combination of an elevated transferrin saturation (>50%) and an elevated ferritin level is 93% sensitive in identifying patients with hemochromatosis. Also, the same combination (elevated transferrin saturation and ferritin level) has a 97% negative predictive accuracy. Thus, in individuals over the age of 35 years, if their transferrin saturation and ferritin are both normal, there is less than a 3% chance that that individual has hemochromatosis.

ii. HFE mutation analysis is recommended within a sibship; thus it will be of benefit here. In a 43-year-old man, the screening iron studies are >97% reliable. Therefore, in the individual described, transferrin saturation and ferritin could be sufficient for screening. Currently, to be more precise, HFE mutation analysis for C282Y and H63D should be performed. This is not only useful within a family, but also it has been proposed by many that genetic testing could very well be utilized in the general population and it is very valuable in a patient with hemochromatosis who has been sporadically identified. HLA-typing is no longer of value in family studies and has never been of value in population screening. If family members are found to be C282Y homozygotes or compound heterozygotes (C282Y/H63D), then they should be considered to have hemochromatosis (provided they have indirect evidence of increased iron stores). If iron studies are abnormal (elevated transferrin saturation or elevated ferritin level) and if the individual is <40 years of age with normal liver enzymes, then it is appropriate to proceed with therapeutic phlebotomy in the absence of a liver biopsy.

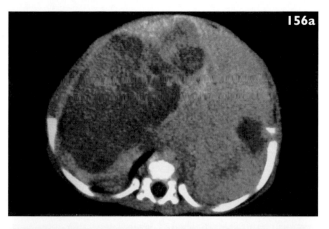

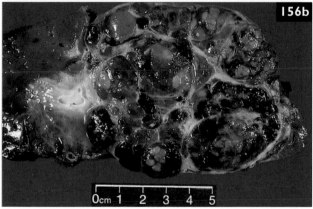

156 A 15-month-old male is noted by his mother to have an enlarging abdomen. His clothes have become tight fitting. He has had a low grade fever and mild anorexia for 2 weeks. On physical examination he has a firm, irregular mass in the right upper quadrant of his abdomen extending across the midline and to the pelvic brim. Laboratory investigations are shown.

Total bilirubin 2.2 mg/dL (37.6 μmol/L)
AST 53 U/L
ALT 335 U/L
ALP 184 U/L
Albumin 3.4 g/dL (34 g/L)
Prothrombin time 14.4 seconds
HBsAg absent
Alphafetoprotein 17,020 ng/mL

i. What do the CT scan (156a) and liver biopsy specimen (156b) from this patient reveal?
ii. What is the likely diagnosis?
iii. What therapy do you recommend?
iv. What is the prognosis?

156 i. The CT scan shows multiple low density lesions throughout the liver of this patient. The cut section of the liver reveals masses scattered throughout that are consistent with a malignant process.

ii. The likely diagnosis based upon the CT scan, pathologic specimen, and clinical history is a hepatoblastoma. Hepatoblastoma is the most common liver tumor in children and is seen usually under 2 years of age. These children often present with an abdominal mass noted by the parents. Hepatoblastoma accounts for about a quarter of all pediatric liver tumors. Half of these are malignant. It is more common in boys than girls and there is no racial predilection. A variety of malformations have been associated with hepatoblastoma. Some of the tumors may produce hormones such as human chorionic gonadotropin. Hepatoblastoma has been associated with Prader–Willi, Beckwith–Wiedemann, and Goldenhar's syndromes. Laboratory studies are usually unremarkable except for a significant elevation of alphafetoprotein. Alphafetoprotein levels may parallel the disease course with diminished levels signifying regression of tumor and elevated levels suggesting tumor growth or metastasis. Imaging studies may be helpful in demonstrating either solitary or multifocal masses with CT attenuation values between water and normal liver parenchyma. Occasionally, calcifications may also be seen in the tumor. Ultrasound examination may reveal a mass with increased, inhomogeneous echogenicity, occasional cystic areas, and calcification. Angiography may demonstrate a hypervascular lesion with distortion and displacement of the vessels. Hepatoblastomas are single masses in 80% of cases with most in the right lobe. They appear coarsely lobulated and may bulge from the liver surface. On cut section, they are often tan or green in color with areas of necrosis and hemorrhage. Histologically, the tumor may be classified into epithelial including fetal, embryonal, macrotrabecular or small cell undifferentiated, and the mixed epithelial and mesenchymal type with or without teratoid features.

iii. Therapy for hepatoblastoma is directed toward resection of the tumor if at all possible. At diagnosis, often 70% of the tumors are unresectable. After chemotherapy, many previously unresectable tumors become potentially resectable. Complete resection of the tumor at the initial laporotomy is the surgical goal of therapy. Liver transplantation, both orthotopic cadaveric and living-related, has also been used successfully in selected cases.

iv. Prognosis for hepatoblastoma is directly related to the presence or absence of metastases at the time of resection. Thus, complete excision of the tumor is the goal of therapy. Overall survival for hepatoblastoma based upon the Children's Cancer Study group experience is about 50%. There is a wide variation in prognosis dependent upon stage. With stage I disease complete tumor resection has an almost 80% survival. Stages III and IV have only about 25% survival.

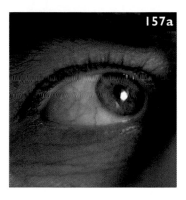

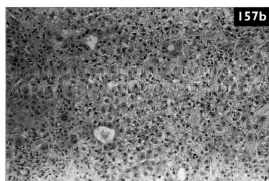

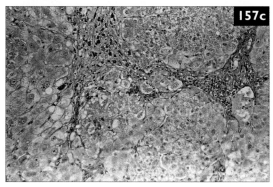

157 A 47-year-old female suffered a traumatic injury with lacerations to her left wrist and hand, requiring a surgical exploration under general anesthesia. Her temperature rose to 101°F (38.3°C) on the day after the operation and subsequently returned to normal. The fever was accompanied by a temporary rise of WBC to 10,200/mm³ (10.2 × 10⁹/L) with eosinophilia. Twelve days after the operation she complained of muscle soreness, nausea, and loss of appetite. On clinical examination she was deeply jaundiced and had no hepatomegaly. Laboratory investigations are shown. A liver biopsy was performed 3 days after admission.

i. Comment on the physical findings shown (157a).
ii. Comment on the liver biopsy findings (157b, c).
iii. What is the diagnosis?
iv. What is the pathogenesis and natural history?
v. Is any specific treatment recommended?

Bilirubin 14.7 mg/dL (251 µmol/L)
ALP 680 U/L
ALT 1,700 U/L
AST 1,250 U/L
BUN 95 mg/dL (urea 15.7 mmol/L)
Albumin 2.9 g/dL (298 g/L)
HBsAg absent
Anti-HCV absent
IgM anti-HAV absent
Anti-liver–kidney microsomal antibodies 1:80
IgM anti-CMV absent
IgM anti-Epstein–Barr virus absent

157 i. Jaundice, due to staining of the tissues with bilirubin, is first detected in the sclera of the eye where it is strongly bound by elastin. Jaundice may be caused by either overproduction (hemolytic anemias) or reduced excretion (liver cell or biliary disease) of bilirubin.

ii. The liver biopsy shows centrilobular necrosis and normal portal tracts. Cholestasis is reflected in dilated bile canaliculi containing bile. Focal necrosis is present (**157b**, H&E). Macrophages are present in the centrilobular area and bridging fibrosis extends toward portal tracts (**157c**, PAS reaction after glycogen digestion).

iii. Halothane induced hepatitis. The spectrum of liver injury that may follow halothane exposure varies from minor increases in serum aminotransferase values to rarer instances of fulminant hepatic failure. Subacute hepatitis, chronic hepatitis, and inactive cirrhosis have been described following halothane hepatitis. The frequency of halothane associated liver damage is estimated to be between 1 in 7,000 and 1 in 30,000. The general criteria for identifying a hypersensitivity reaction are: the presence of a sensitization period, prompt recurrence of liver disease on re-exposure, association with rash, fever, and eosinophilia. Occasionally there may be a blood dyscrasia or liver granulomata.

iv. Halothane is transformed by cytochrome P450 in two ways. The reductive pathway leads to a free radical that can initiate lipid peroxidation and might be responsible for the subclinical increase in serum aminotransferase activity observed in a number of patients. The oxidative pathway leads to a trifluoroacetyl chloride intermediate which covalently binds to the amino groups of proteins. Previous exposure of patients to these metabolites may lead to a more severe form of halothane hepatitis injury. These patients have all the features of an immunoallergic reaction with fever, eosinophilia, and nonorgan-specific autoantibodies including anti-liver-kidney microsomal antibodies. Such patients may have a high incidence of antibodies to both normal liver cell components and specifically to halothane related antigens. In addition, they show a high incidence of histocompatibility antigens A11 and BW22. The mean interval between exposure and onset of jaundice is 12 days after a first exposure and reduces progressively as the number of previous exposures increases. With few exceptions, halothane induced hepatitis does not proceed to chronicity. In a few patients inactive cirrhosis may persist. The mortality is about 40% in patients developing jaundice.

v. Uncomplicated cases of halothane hepatitis require supporting measures and careful monitoring. Patients developing fulminant hepatic failure may be successfully treated with liver transplantation. Drug induced injury was the primary indication in 9.6% of all fulminant hepatitis cases in children and 16% of all cases in adults undergoing liver transplantation in the USA.

158 A 68-year-old male on warfarin for chronic atrial fibrillation with a previously stable, therapeutic prothrombin time returns from a month long cruise. Other than a 10 lb (4.5 kg) weight gain which the patient attributes to dietary overindulgence including heavy alcohol use, the patient feels well. The patient adamantly claims to have been compliant with his warfarin therapy. However, his prothrombin time is prolonged outside his normal therapeutic range.
i. How does the patient's alcohol use affect his response to warfarin therapy?
ii. What other commonly used drugs does alcohol alter in a similar manner?
iii. How else might alcohol alter drug responses?

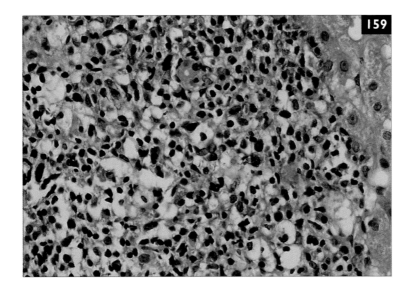

159 A patient who underwent liver transplantation 6 months ago develops chills at night and adenopathy in the neck. His WBC count is low and his biochemical liver test results are normal. A scalene node is biopsied (159).
i. What is the differential diagnosis and the most likely explanation?
ii. What are the treatment options for this patient and how would you decide which to employ?

158 i. The microsomal induction resulting from long term alcohol consumption increases the metabolism of other microsomal substrates, including warfarin. As a result, the warfarin is more rapidly metabolized, resulting in a subtherapeutic prothrombin time.

ii. Phenytoin, tolbutamide, propranolol, rifampicin, meprobamate, pentobarbitol, methadone, and barbiturates administration alter warfarin metabolism. In the setting of chronic alcoholism, increased metabolism and tolerance is commonly encountered.

iii. In the presence of alcohol intoxication, the opposite effect (greater therapeutic response) may result because of competition with the drug for microsomal oxidation. As a result, there may be dangerously high levels in the blood. In addition, the normal metabolism of drugs may be altered, producing toxicity. Drug hepatotoxicity, e.g. isoniazid and methotrexate, is also increased. Cytochrome P450 activation leads to a greater production of carcinogens from procarcinogens, partly accounting for the association of alcoholism with an increased incidence of various cancers.

159 i. The symptoms described here are nonspecific and may represent either a generalized infection or a process such as PTLD. The patient has generalized lymphadenopathy, which could represent tuberculosis in a transplant patient. However, the low WBC count is inconsistent with tuberculosis and the biopsy shown above has no granulomas. Rather, the biopsy shows the typical picture of PTLD. The lymph node architecture is distorted, and there is an abundance of atypical lymphocytes replacing the node. PTLD arises in the setting of intense immunosuppression and is thought to result from disruption of the ability of the normal immune system to perform surveillance against the development of neoplastic cells. It is almost always associated with Epstein–Barr virus infection and the use of immunosuppressive agents. The exact pathogenesis is unclear, but PTLD is usually a polyclonal process. It can involve the transplanted organ and the lymph nodes or can present with single organ involvement, such as with bleeding or perforation in the gastrointestinal tract. One half of 1% of all transplant patients are affected with this disease.

ii. Treatment of PTLD depends on the presentation and the clonality of the tumor. A common denominator of therapy must be withdrawal of immunosuppression, to the extent possible. In the case of nonlifesaving organ transplants such as the kidney, the immunosuppression can be completely withdrawn and the organ can be sacrificed. With lifesaving organs such as the heart, lungs, and liver, a delicate balance between the withdrawal of immunosuppression and the development of rejection of the transplanted organ must be reached. When the disease is polyclonal, withdrawal of immunosuppression alone may be sufficient treatment. In some instances, agents such as ganciclovir and intravenous Ig are added to decrease the viral load. Alpha-interferon, a nonspecific immunostimulant, has also been used for this purpose. When the tumor is monoclonal, the response rates to this treatment are lower, as are the survival rates. Most experts favor the additional use of systemic chemotherapy in this instance.

160 A 2-month-old male born at 32 weeks gestation has spent his life in the neonatal intensive care unit. Initially, he had respiratory distress and required ventilator support for 2 weeks. He has been unable to take oral feeds and has a central venous catheter through which he has received TPN. Recently, the neonatal intensive care nurses have noticed that he appears jaundiced. Laboratory investigations are shown.

What is the likely diagnosis?

Total bilirubin 8.5 mg/dL (145.35 µmol/L)
Direct-reacting bilirubin 5.2 mg/dL
(88.9 µmol/L)
AST 175 U/L
ALT 177 U/L
ALT 177 U/L

161 A 48-year-old female patient with alcoholic cirrhosis does well for 4 months following endoscopic band ligation of varices but then returns with another episode of endoscopically documented esophageal variceal hemorrhage. On this occasion, two attempts at controlling the bleeding, 24 hours apart, are unsuccessful. The patient is given 6 units of blood and continues to pass maroon colored stools. A TIPS is placed and she has no further bleeding (**161**). After some early postoperative encephalopathy which responded readily to treatment with lactulose, the patient remains abstinent from alcohol for the next 8 months and is able to return to work. Within the last month, however, she

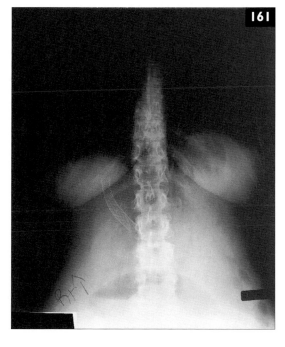

has noted an increase in abdominal girth and now presents with a 1 day history of melena. Endoscopy reveals esophageal varices as the source of bleeding. She responds to initial measures to control the bleeding. A Doppler ultrasound reveals a thrombosed TIPS which is confirmed by angiography.

i. What initial maneuvers are instituted by the therapeutic radiologist?
ii. What longer term options would you consider?

160 TPN related liver disease is the likely diagnosis. TPN associated liver disease is the most common nutrition related liver disorder. In infants, cholestasis is the typical response observed. There may be biliary sludge, cholelithiasis, and development of fibrosis and cirrhosis over time. In infants, cholestasis may be insidious. Clinically, hepatomegaly on physical examination may be followed by biochemical evidence of cholestasis (elevated serum bile acid levels or direct-reacting bilirubin). Serum aminotransferase and ALP levels increase but this may occur many days to weeks later. At increased risk for the development of TPN associated liver disease are premature infants and infants exclusively receiving parenteral nutrition without any enteral nutrition. The diagnosis of TPN associated liver disease is one of exclusion. The pathogenesis of TPN associated liver disease is unknown but probably multi-factorial. These infants often have variable periods of starvation caused by the inability to use the gastrointestinal tract, mucosal injury, bacterial overgrowth, and so on. These infants also often have episodes of hypoxia and hypotension which contribute to hepatic injury. Additionally, infants have inefficient ability for bile salt uptake, intrahepatocyte transport and processing, and canalicular excretion. This 'physiologic' immaturity is related to an immaturity of perinatal metabolic pathways within the liver. A lack of enteral feeds also appears to be an important contributing factor in the severity of the hepatic pathology observed. Starvation results in diminished gastrointestinal hormone secretion with resultant decreased intestinal motility, decreased bile flow, and impaired mucosal immunity.

161 i. Although late shunt occlusions tend to be more resistant to balloon dilation than stenotic shunts without occlusion, the initial approach for the occluded shunt is balloon dilation. If this is unsuccessful, a second parallel TIPS is inserted to achieve adequate portal decompression.

ii. This patient has now been abstinent for 8 months. She has had a second episode of variceal hemorrhage because of TIPS malfunction. Although she may temporarily be controlled by correction of the shunt malfunction, she should be considered for liver transplantation at this point. In a meta-analysis of eight randomized controlled trials comparing TIPS with sclerotherapy for the prevention of variceal rebleeding, 18.2% of patients treated with TIPS rebled compared to 42.1% receiving sclerotherapy. A survey involving 1,750 patients treated with TIPS reported stenosis or occlusion in 92% of patients experiencing an episode of variceal rebleeding. In a prospective evaluation of 100 consecutive patients treated with TIPS and followed for a mean of 1,050 days a cumulative incidence of recurrent portal hypertension of 90% at 2 years as measured by an increase in portal pressure was reported. Despite early detection and treatment of stent dysfunction, portal hypertension recurred within the majority of patients during the initial year after the TIPS placement. In a long term follow-up of patients treated with TIPS, a cumulative rebleeding rate of 26% at 1 year and 32% at 2 years was reported. This rebleeding rate occurred despite very careful follow-up and vigorous attempts to treat the stent dysfunction. TIPS should be considered a short to intermediate term treatment for prevention of recurrent variceal bleeding until the problem of stent dysfunction is solved.

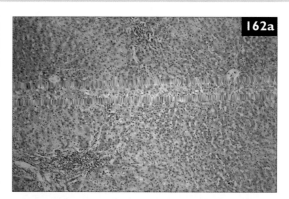

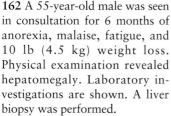

CBC normal
Bilirubin 0.4 mg/dL (6.84 μmol/L)
ESR 46 mm/hour
Total protein 7.3 g/dL (73 g/L)
GGT 200 U/L
Albumin 3.4 g/dL (34 g/L)
AST 29 U/L
ALP 268 U/L

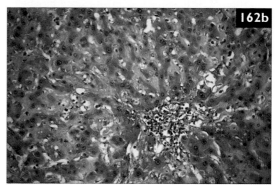

162 A 55-year-old male was seen in consultation for 6 months of anorexia, malaise, fatigue, and 10 lb (4.5 kg) weight loss. Physical examination revealed hepatomegaly. Laboratory investigations are shown. A liver biopsy was performed.
i. Describe the biopsy findings shown (**162a**).
ii. Describe the biopsy findings shown (**162b**).
iii. What is the diagnosis?
iv. Biopsies of what other tissues might yield a diagnosis?
v. Describe the clinical features of this condition.

163 A 23-year-old gravida 1, para 1, white female presents for evaluation of abnormal iron studies. At the time of a routine postpartum visit, a screening chemistry panel included a transferrin saturation that was elevated at 80%. A follow-up repeat fasting transferrin saturation was again elevated at 75%, and the serum ferritin level was increased at 420 ng/mL (7.5 μmol/L). Her CBC and blood chemistry studies were normal. There is no family history of liver disease or of hemochromatosis. The patient feels well except for some fatigue. Physical examination is normal.
i. Is it possible that a young woman of childbearing age could have phenotypic evidence of hemochromatosis?
ii. Should this patient have a liver biopsy?
iii. If a liver biopsy is undertaken and there is only a slight increase in hepatic iron concentration, how can you tell whether or not this patient has hemochromatosis?

162 i. This low power view of the liver (**162a**) shows infiltration of sinusoids with an amorphous homogenous pale material compatible with amyloid.

ii. The biopsy findings on this Congo red stain show the same sinusoidal deposition of amyloid. Not shown on this biopsy is the pattern of amyloid deposition in the hepatic artery and portal vein.

iii. The diagnosis is systemic amyloidosis, which may occur as a primary/myeloma-related condition, as a secondary/reactive condition, or as a familial form. Hepatic involvement in all three major forms of systemic amyloidosis is common.

iv. Biopsies of gingiva, rectum, or abdominal fat may all be used to make a diagnosis. The abdominal fat aspiration technique is often employed because it is safe and can be easily performed at the bedside.

v. Clinical evidence of liver dysfunction is often minor. There may be only a slight elevation of ALP and, or, GGT noted on biochemical profile, with mild hepatomegaly on physical examination. Primary or myeloma-related systemic amyloidosis often occurs in association with plasma cell dyscrasias or in association with heavy chain disease. Secondary or reactive systemic amyloidosis occurs in the presence of a number of long standing chronic inflammatory processes.

163 i. Recent studies have identified young women with hereditary hemochromatosis: studies that have relied on either family screening or on the use of transferrin saturation on screening chemistry panels have shown a male to female ratio of about 2:1. This still underestimates the genotypic expression of hemochromatosis, which has a male to female ratio of 1:1.

ii. As the transferrin saturation and ferritin levels are both elevated, HFE mutation analysis should be performed (see **155**); this combination is highly sensitive and specific for hereditary hemochromatosis. A liver biopsy is not indicated with normal liver function tests.

iii. The calculated hepatic iron index is particularly helpful in young individuals. When individuals with homozygous hereditary hemochromatosis are identified at a young age, their degree of iron-loading is often not very high but their hepatic iron concentration will be increased above the upper limit of normal. Individuals like this will often have hepatic iron concentrations in the 3,000 to 6,000 µg/g (dry weight) range. Use of the hepatic iron index, which is the hepatic iron concentration in µmol/g dry weight divided by the patient's age, accommodates for a lower iron concentration at a younger age. In fact, it is based on the principle that in homozygotes, iron deposition is progressive with age. In heterozygotes or in individuals with mild secondary iron overload related to some other underlying liver disease, the iron concentration is not progressive with age. Therefore, taking the hepatic iron concentration and dividing by age allows for a differentiation between homozygous hereditary hemochromatosis patients, heterozygotes, and patients with mild secondary iron overload. In this patient the hepatic iron concentration was 6,350 µg/g dry weight which gives a concentration of 113.4 µmol/g dry weight. This value is then divided by the patient's age in years (23 years) which gives an hepatic iron index of 4.9 which is above the cut-off value of 1.9. Therefore, this individual definitely has homozygous hereditary hemochromatosis.

164 A 10-year-old white male is hospitalized with abdominal pain, nausea, and malaise of 8 weeks duration. His past history included a seizure disorder, for which he has received valproic acid 250 mg four times a day for the past 6 months and phenytoin 400 mg every day for the past 2 years. Twenty-four hours after admission, lethargy, anorexia, vomiting, and increased convulsions are observed, and are followed subsequently by jaundice, ascites, and coma. Laboratory investigations are shown. A liver biopsy is performed which reveals extensive microvesicular steatosis and centrilobular necrosis.

AST 280 U/L
ALT 120 U/L
Bilirubin 4.2 mg/dL (71.8 µmol/L)
ALP 270 U/l
Albumin 4.6 g/dL (46 g/L)
Prothrombin time 14 seconds
Glucose 28 mg/dL (1.5 mmol/L)
Blood ammonia 105 µg/dL (61.6 µmol/L)
HBsAg, anti-HBs, IgM anti-HBc, IgM anti-HAV, and anti-HCV absent
Alpha-1-antitrypsin, ceruloplasmin, and ferritin levels normal

i. What is the most likely diagnosis?
ii. What is the pathogenesis of this condition?
iii. What is the management of this condition?

165 A 6-year-old child underwent a liver biopsy in the evaluation of suspected Reye's syndrome. Both light and electron microscope evaluation are helpful in assessing patients with suspected Reye's syndrome. Liver histology reveals a characteristic severe fatty infiltration with small droplet fat (microvesicular) with notable absence of inflammation. Fat stains readily demonstrate the droplets as in the present case. Ultrastructural studies of hepatocytes using electron microscopy reveal significantly altered mitochondria. Histochemical staining reveals a striking depletion of the mitochondrial enzyme succinic dehydrogenase.

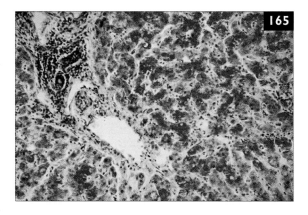

i. Comment on the liver biopsy (**165**).
ii. What is the recommended treatment?
iii. What is the prognosis for children following recovery from Reye's syndrome?

164 i. Valproic hepatotoxicity. In this patient, liver failure can be reasonably attributed to valproic acid mainly because of the time interval between drug administration (6 months) and the subsequent development of hepatic failure characterized histologically by microvesicular steatosis and centrilobular necrosis. Other findings supportive of this etiology include the absence of clinical, biochemical or histological evidence of previous chronic liver disease and the reasonable exclusion of viral etiology by serologic tests and history. Microvesicular steatosis is a histological pattern of liver injury characteristic of a select group of drugs and toxins that includes valproic acid, tetracycline, and hypoglycin. It is also encountered in the setting of inborn and acquired disorders of fatty acid oxidation that include Reye's syndrome, and acute fatty liver of pregnancy.
ii. Valproic acid is a branched chain fatty acid. Its metabolites inhibit mitochondrial beta oxidation of long chain fatty acids. Coenzyme A derivatives of valproic acid accumulate as well and the resultant depletion in hepatocellular levels of coenzyme A may also serve to impair normal oxidative fatty acid metabolism. Intrahepatic accumulation of fatty acids results in increased triglyceride synthesis and the microvesicular fatty change while reduced ATP production may contribute to deranged liver function.
iii. There is no effective treatment for valproic acid hepatotoxicity, but spontaneous recovery is the rule after discontinuation of the drug. Oral carnitine has been suggested to prevent or ameliorate the toxicity, but its effectiveness is unproven.

165 i. This is an oil red O-stained section of liver revealing an extensive accumulation of small fat droplets in the cytoplasm of hepatocytes that do not displace the nucleus. There is some coalescence of fat droplets to form larger sized droplets. Inflammation and necrosis of parenchyma are not evident. Small droplet fat (microvesicular) on liver biopsy is associated with Reye's syndrome, with tetracycline hepatotoxicity, and with acute fatty liver of pregnancy.
ii. Treatment for Reye's syndrome is mostly supportive. Successful treatment is dependent upon: an early and accurate diagnosis using liver biopsy and lumbar puncture, vigilant clinical observation, early and elective endotracheal intubation and placement of central lines for monitoring, continuous intravenous glucose administration, and maintenance of normal intravascular volume to prevent hypoglycemia and hypovolemia. Glucose infusion has been found to be an important component of Reye's syndrome therapy and provides a substrate for lost glycogen stores, halts lipolysis, and provides plasma hyperosmolarity. Elevated intracranial pressure is not the cause of coma seen in Reye's syndrome, but it can be responsible for significant morbidity and mortality.
iii. Following recovery from Reye's syndrome, children may have short term cognitive deficits and may require adjustments in their school program. The long term prognosis is good with most children recovering completely. If sequelae occur, they are usually the result of complications such as hypoglycemia, hypoxia, hypotension, and uncontrolled intracranial hypertension. Recurrent Reye's syndrome probably does not exist. A recurrence of symptoms should prompt an evaluation for a possible metabolic defect, especially involving the urea cycle or fatty acid oxidation.

166 A 53-year-old male presented with jaundice, fatigue, and hepatomegaly. These symptoms developed 3 days after onset of dark urine, fever, and chills. He denied alcohol abuse and exposure to risk factors for viral hepatitis. However, 6 weeks before disease onset he visited North Africa. Laboratory investigations are shown. Abdominal ultrasound shows a moderately enlarged liver and normal spleen.

Bilirubin 14.5 mg/dL (248 µmol/L)
ALT 2,640 U/L
AST 2,200 U/L
HBsAg absent
Anti-HCV absent
IgM anti-HAV present
Prothrombin time 16 seconds
Platelet count 240,000/mm³ (240 × 10⁹/L)

i. What is diagnosis? What is the clinical presentation of this condition?
ii. What is the epidemiology and natural history of the disease?

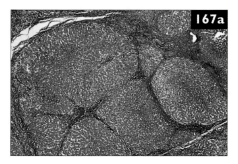

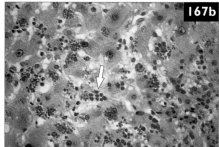

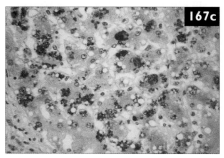

167 A 63-year-old female was admitted to the hospital with acute esophageal variceal bleeding. She underwent emergency endoscopic band ligation. Her recurrent hemorrhage could not be controlled leading to exsanguination and death. There had been no known personal or family history of liver disease. An autopsy was performed.

i. Describe the trichrome stain slide (**167a**).
ii. Describe the findings on this high power PAS with diastase stain (**167b**, arrow).
iii. Describe the findings on immunoperoxidase staining (**167c**).
iv. What is the diagnosis and pathophysiology of this condition?
v. What tests are useful to make a diagnosis before biopsy?

166 i. The diagnosis is acute infection with hepatitis A virus, a small RNA virus belonging to the picornavirus family. The diagnosis rests on detection of serum IgM antibody to hepatitis A virus. IgG antibody to hepatitis A virus indicates recovery and specific immunity against hepatitis A virus. IgM antibody is almost invariably found at onset of symptoms or 1 week later, and may persist for months. The clinical picture of hepatitis A differs according to the patient's age. Jaundice is unusual in infants, whereas symptomatic, icteric, hepatitis is common in adults. Fulminant hepatitis A occurs in 1% of patients above the age of 50.

ii. Transmission of hepatitis A virus is almost invariably by the fecal–oral route. However, as viremia precedes the onset of jaundice by several weeks, occasional transmission of virus through blood donations or clotting factor concentrates occurs. Commonly reported risk factors among patients with hepatitis A are household exposure, contacts with children in day care, male homosexual activity, illicit drug abuse, and visiting areas which are endemic for hepatitis A virus. Unlike hepatitis B virus and hepatitis C virus, hepatitis A viral infection does not carry the risk of chronic infection. Liver injury in hepatitis A is invariably transient, although a small number of patients may develop a self-limited form of relapsing hepatitis. A few patients may also develop prolonged (6–12 months) cholestatic hepatitis, characterized by jaundice and pruritus.

167 i. This low magnification view of a trichrome stained slide shows a macronodular cirrhosis with bands of fibrous tissue surrounding hepatocytes which appear to have prominent cytoplasmic staining.

ii. This high magnification of a PAS with diastase stained slide shows intensely stained PAS-positive globules within the cytoplasm. This is the classic finding of homozygous alpha-1-antitrypsin deficiency in individuals with the PiZZ phenotype, i.e. PAS-positive, diastase-resistant globules in periportal hepatocytes. Although these globules are readily seen on H&E staining, they are most prominent on a PAS with diastase stain.

iii. Immunoperoxidase staining for the abnormal glycoprotein of alpha-1-antitrypsin is also useful in confirming the diagnosis.

iv. The diagnosis is homozygous alpha-1-antitrypsin deficiency. The pathophysiology involves a single amino acid substitution which leads to synthesis of an abnormal protein that can not be secreted and accumulates in the endoplasmic reticulum. Liver injury results from accumulation of this abnormal alpha-1-antitrypsin molecule. Patients with PiZZ homozygous alpha-1-antitrypsin deficiency may have neonatal hepatitis, childhood cirrhosis, adult chronic hepatitis, cirrhosis, or hepatocellular carcinoma. The outcome is variable and there may be a long period of minimal hepatic dysfunction before progression to cirrhosis.

v. The diagnosis is best made by determination of the alpha-1-antitrypsin phenotype. Patients have a decrease in the serum alpha-1-antitrypsin level, which is found to be <50% of normal in patients with homozygous disease. Liver biopsy with detection of the characteristic PAS-positive diastase-resistant cytoplasmic globules is confirmatory.

168 A 19-year-old female, previously an honors student in school, could no longer concentrate on schoolwork. She became withdrawn and complained of insomnia. After several months, she noted difficulty with her speech and an uncontrollable tremor of her hands. She was referred to a neurologist who noted splenomegaly. Laboratory investigations showed elevated serum aminotransferase activities and a normal serum ceruloplasmin of 220 mg/L. A CT scan of her brain showed bilateral basal ganglia lesions, prompting a slit-lamp examination which revealed Kayser–Fleischer rings. A liver biopsy was subsequently performed and she was noted to have cirrhosis, a positive Rhodanine histochemical staining, and a quantitative hepatic copper of 750 µg/g dry weight liver. She was started on penicillamine and over the next week developed a fever and rash. Her platelet count was noted to decrease from 90 to 33 × 10³/mm³ (× 10⁹/L). The penicillamine was withdrawn and she was placed on trientine dihydrochloride. The neurologic changes remained unchanged over the next few weeks, however, she was noted to become progressively anemic and depressed.

i. What is her diagnosis?

ii. What is the possible cause of the developing anemia? What alternative treatment should be considered?

169 A 27-year-old female underwent laparoscopic chole-cystectomy for biliary colic. An ultrasound scan had shown three stones within a nonfunc-tioning gallbladder. The bile duct was not visualized. Bio-chemical liver tests showed mild elevation of ALP activity. Laparoscopic cholecystectomy was difficult because of severe inflammation and adhesions. The patient was readmitted 5 days after the procedure with pleural effusion, abdominal pain, and jaundice.

i. What does this ERCP show (**169**)?

ii. What treatment is indicated?

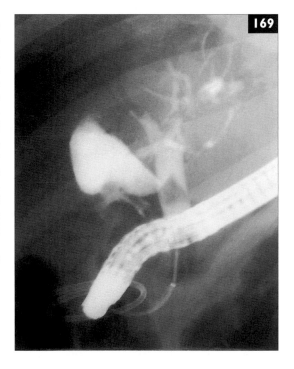

168 i. This patient manifested mainly psychiatric and neurologic manifestations of Wilson's disease. Patients who present with these symptoms are typically older than those presenting with hepatic signs or symptoms. It is not uncommon to find a significant period of time between onset of symptoms and disease recognition and treatment. This is due to the non-distinctive initial manifestations. This patient had a normal level of serum ceruloplasmin which can occur in about 5% of patients with Wilson's disease and which can delay the continued search to exclude this disorder. The presence of Kayser–Fleischer rings, the elevated hepatic copper, and positive Rhodanine histochemistry for copper binding protein confirms the diagnosis of Wilson's disease.

ii. The development of anemia while on trientine therapy is thought to be caused by the removal of copper from marrow stores which results in the failure to correctly mobilize iron. This can be recognized on marrow examination by the presence of sideroblasts. This is one of the few side effects of trientine, and is resolved by discontinuation of this drug. One therapeutic option for this symptomatic patient is to reinstitute penicillamine treatment using a desensitization protocol. Progressive dosages of the penicillamine are administered with corticosteroid therapy which can be withdrawn over time. Another is to use the alternative agent zinc which acts to reduce copper absorption by the gut and places patients in negative copper balance. The experience with zinc for symptomatic patients is limited, and this agent is probably best used adjunctively or on asymptomatic patients for maintenance therapy. Another experimental treatment for neurologic Wilson's disease is tetra-thiomolybdate, an alternative chelating agent.

169 i. The ERCP shows a dilated common bile duct associated with a calculus. In addition contrast is leaking from the area of the cystic stump into the peritoneal cavity beneath the liver. A previously inserted percutaneous drain is also seen on this radiograph. It is likely that in this case the clip positioned on the cystic duct was inadequately placed. The pressure within the biliary system was high as a consequence of the bile duct calculus and both factors combined to cause a biliary leak. Bile duct injury occurs more commonly after laparoscopy than after open cholecystectomy. It is also more frequent with inexperienced surgeons and in the presence of adhesions within the gallbladder bed.

ii. The treatment of choice is to remove the bile duct calculus by balloon or basket extraction after sphincterotomy and insertion of a plastic stent across the cystic duct defect. The stent is removed 4–6 weeks later. This results in the cystic duct stump spontaneously closing, stopping the leak. Open laparotomy with surgical repair remains an option.

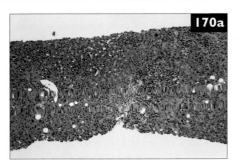 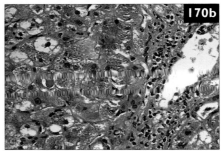

170a Although liver biopsy is not generally needed in patients with acute hepatitis, the histologic features may be indicative of acute hepatocyte injury.

i. What features of this biopsy specimen are characteristic of acute viral hepatitis (**170a, b**)?

ii. This patient was found to have hepatitis A. Can this disease be prevented?

171 A 50-year-old male was admitted because of nausea and abdominal malaise of 3 days duration. The past medical history revealed that he had been admitted 8 years previously because of ascites attributed to alcoholic liver cirrhosis. On this admission his temperature was 100.3°F (37.9°C) and his abdomen was distended with ascites but without tenderness. The peripheral WBC count was 13,000/mm³ (13 × 10⁹/L) with 90% polymorphonuclear cells. Urinalysis

First paracentesis
Total nucleated cells 700/mm³ (7 × 10⁸/L)
   (80% polymorphonuclears)
Protein 1.5 g/dL (15 g/L)
Glucose 95 mg/dL (5.27 mmol/L)

Second paracentesis
Total nucleated cells 900/mm³ (9 × 10⁸/L)
   (75% polymorphonuclears)
Protein 1.7 g/dL (17 g/L)
Glucose 89 mg/dL (4.94 mmol/L)

revealed 20–30 WBC per high-power field and a few bacteria. The laboratory results of a paracentesis are shown. The patient was diagnosed with spontaneous bacterial peritonitis and placed on intravenous cefotaxime. Because of a temperature spike to 100.4°F (38°C) and after 4 days of treatment, a second paracentesis was performed and the results are shown.

i. What do the results of the first ascitic fluid sample reveal?

ii. Comment on the polymorphonuclear count after the initiation of therapy. What is the most likely diagnosis?

iii. Which other investigations would you perform?

170 i. The liver biopsy shows preserved lobular architecture, and lymphohistiocytic infiltration of the portal tracts. There is slight piecemeal necrosis at the borders of portal tracts and focal intralobular inflammation (170a). Peculiar features of acute liver cell necrosis during viral hepatitis include acidophilic bodies ballooning liver cells, and edema (170b).

ii. Yes. Infection can be prevented short term with 0.02 mL/kg human IgG given intramuscularly either after exposure or pre-exposure. Post-exposure prophylaxis is recommended for intrafamily or sexual contacts, or persons resident or working in an institution where a case of hepatitis A developed. Pre-exposure prophylaxis is indicated to protect travellers to endemic areas and military personnel. Vaccination can confer long term immunity against hepatitis A virus and is recommended for all the above cited persons, with the adjunct of food handlers, homosexuals, health care workers, and patients with liver disease. Patients with asymptomatic or mild forms of hepatitis A do not need special care other than observation. Those with symptoms may be treated with bed rest, a light diet, and closer surveillance. Intravenous fluids, glucose, and salts can be given to those patients who have nausea, loss of appetite, or vomiting. Fulminant hepatic failure caused by hepatitis A virus has successfully been treated with liver transplantation.

171 i. In view of an ascitic fluid with more than 250 polymorphonuclear leukocytes with normal proteins, and glucose, the initial diagnosis of spontaneous bacterial peritonitis seems straightforward. In this setting the possibility of gut perforation is unlikely.

ii. The polymorphonuclear count in ascitic fluid usually decreases exponentially in spontaneous bacterial peritonitis once antibiotic treatment is initiated, with <50% of the initial value after 48 hours. The lack of such a rapid decline is strong evidence against spontaneous peritonitis and in favor of secondary peritonitis. In this case it would probably correspond to a nonperforation type of secondary peritonitis (e.g. loculated perforation of a peptic ulcer, infected pancreatic pseudocyst, perinephric abscess, acute appendicitis). These conditions are not readily apparent on the basis of the initial ascitic fluid analysis and should be considered in view of the response of the cell count and cultures to treatment.

iii. Barium enema, gastrointestinal X-ray series, and abdominal CT or ultrasound should be used in order to localize the primary site of infection. In this case an abdominal ultrasound showed a perinephric abscess which was drained percutaneously.

172 A 48-year-old male, known to be infected with hepatitis B and D viruses, was referred to the liver unit for upper gastrointestinal bleeding. Endoscopy revealed bleeding esophageal varices which were treated with band ligation.

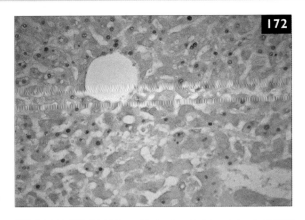

Laboratory investigations are shown. Ultrasound examination revealed a reduced liver size and no evidence of hepatocellular carcinoma. During admission he developed tense ascites which rapidly became unresponsive to diuretic therapy. Six months later the patient underwent liver transplantation.

i. Was the patient a good candidate for liver transplantation?

ii. Did the patient need any treatment to prevent reinfection?

AST 25 U/L
ALT 38 U/L
Prothrombin time 68 seconds
Albumin 2.2 g/dL (22 g/L)
Hemoglobin 8.5 g/dL (85 g/L)
WBC count 2,400/mm³ (2.4 × 10⁹/L)
Platelet count 42,000/mm³ (42 × 10⁹/L)
HBsAg present, IgM anti-HBc absent, HBeAg absent, hepatitis B virus-DNA absent
Anti-HD present, IgM anti-HD present (titer: 10⁻²), hepatitis D virus-RNA absent
Anti-HCV absent

iii. One month after liver transplantation the patient underwent a liver biopsy. Despite only mildly elevated liver enzymes and negative hepatitis B virus serum markers, the liver biopsy showed positive staining for hepatitis D antigens in several nuclei, no staining for HBsAg and HBcAg, and mild degenerative lesions of the hepatocytes (**172**). Is this finding compatible with the obligatory helper function of hepatitis B virus for hepatitis D virus infection?

iv. Six months after liver transplantation the patient developed an episode of acute hepatitis. Which is the most likely etiology of the acute episode?

v. If the patient becomes reinfected what is the prognosis? What is the best available treatment to prevent progression of the hepatitis D virus recurrence?

173 Gilbert's syndrome is commonly suspected in asymptomatic individuals. What diagnostic tests have been proposed to confirm the diagnosis of this condition? Is a liver biopsy indicated in the evaluation of a person with suspected Gilbert's syndrome?

172 i. Liver transplantation provides a valid treatment for end-stage hepatitis D virus disease. As with other viral disorders, transplantation is aggravated by the risk of reinfection, but this is lower for hepatitis D virus than for hepatitis B and C viruses. The clinical course of recurrent hepatitis is milder than for hepatitis B virus.

ii. The patient was transplanted in the early years of the transplantation era and received only 3 months prophylactic treatment with anti-HBs. The prospect of an uneventful clinical course after transplantation can be further improved by long term administration of hyperimmune serum against HBsAg. The 5 year survival rate of 76 hepatitis D virus transplant patients in Paris was 88% with reappearance of HBsAg in only 9% under long term anti-HBs prophylaxis.

iii. Following liver transplantation hepatitis D may establish subclinical and sub-biochemical infection independently of an overt hepatitis B virus infection suggesting that the co-operation with hepatitis B virus is not mandatory for hepatitis D viral reinfection.

iv. The episode of acute hepatitis was associated with serum markers of hepatitis B viral infection and replication. The histological pattern changed from mild degenerative lesions to severe necroinflammation with stainable HBsAg, HBcAg, and HDAg. Hepatitis B virus reactivation did, therefore, trigger a full blown hepatitis recurrence. This event occurs in up to 80% of hepatitis D virus transplanted patients if they are not adequately protected with anti-HBs prophylaxis. Evaluation of the use of lamivudine and other antivirals is on going.

v. So far no treatment has proved to be effective against hepatitis D virus reinfection. Interferon is ineffective and can potentially trigger the rejection of the graft. No data are at present available for lamivudine, a nucleic acid analogue which in hepatitis B virus transplanted patients is highly effective in preventing or treating reinfection.

173 The tests that have been proposed to confirm the diagnosis of Gilbert's syndrome include calorie restriction, the intravenous infusion or the oral administration of nicotinic acid, and the administration of enzyme-inducing agents. Although calorie restriction worsens the hyperbilirubinemia of Gilbert's syndrome, fasting induces hyperbilirubinemia in the general population, thus, this method does not allow for the establishment of an unequivocal diagnosis. Nicotinic acid administration (oral or intravenous) results in an increase in osmotic fragility of RBCs leading to an increase in their sequestration by the spleen. This in turn results in an increased destruction of RBCs and increased production of bilirubin. Phenobarbital administration is associated with normalization of elevated bilirubin levels in this syndrome, as well as an increase in the clearance of hepatic bilirubin. However, the activity of hepatic bilirubin uridine diphosphate-glucuronyltransferase activity has not been found to be increased by phenobarbital in *in vitro* assays in all subjects studied. Interestingly, prednisone administration may decrease the hyperbilirubinemia of Gilbert's syndrome. A follow-up period (e.g. 2 years) of these patients is prudent to confirm the diagnosis. Liver biopsy is not indicated because no substantial abnormalities will be found and it will not be diagnostic.

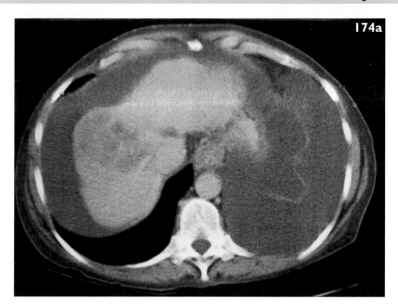

174 A 72-year-old Caucasian male presented with increasing abdominal girth of 3 months duration. The patient has a long history of alcohol abuse, but denies prior gastrointestinal bleeding or confusion. Physical examination was notable for abdominal distension, shifting dullness, and moderate splenomegaly. The liver was ballotable and not enlarged.

Laboratory investigations are shown.

Platelet count 82,000/mm³ (82 × 10⁹/L)
Albumin 2.8 g/dL (28 g/L)
ALT 55 U/L
AST 65 U/L
Total bilirubin 1.2 mg/dL (20.5 µmol/L)
Creatinine 1.3 mg/dL (114.9 µmol/L)
Prothrombin time 14.5 seconds
HBsAg, anti-HBc, and anti-HCV tests absent
Serum alphafetoprotein 7,550 ng/mL

Abdominal ultrasound and CT scans showed a 7 cm (2.7 in) mass in the right liver near the porta hepatis (**174a**). The liver was decreased in size and nodular in appearance. Moderate ascites and splenomegaly were noted. The portal vein was patent and no adenopathy was detected. Chest X-ray showed no infiltrates or nodules.

i. What is the diagnosis in this patient?

ii. What treatment options should be considered?

174 i. A diagnosis of hepatocellular carcinoma is made in this patient based on the markedly elevated serum alphafetoprotein level in association with a hepatic mass in a cirrhotic liver.

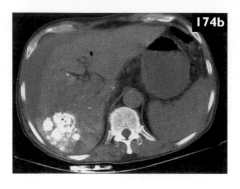

ii. This patient is not considered a candidate for hepatic resection because of an estimation of inadequate hepatic reserve. The liver is cirrhotic with impaired synthetic function and the tumor is located in a position which requires a large proportion of the liver to be removed during resection. A number of treatment modalities are currently available for the treatment of nonresectable hepatocellular carcinoma which is localized to the liver. Intrahepatic arterial chemotherapy with embolization (chemoembolization) can be administered by subselective catheterization of hepatic arterial branches supplying the neoplasm without adversely affecting the nontumorous liver (174b). The vascular supply of hepatocellular carcinoma is predominantly from the hepatic artery. Occlusion of arterial branches can be obtained without significant toxicity as the nontumorous liver can still receive blood from the portal vein. A patent portal vein with normal directional flow is, therefore, a requirement in patients treated with chemoembolization. Tumor necrosis can be accomplished in up to 70% of patients treated with chemo-embolization. However, the treatment is considered palliative because of the frequent finding of residual viable tumor cells, particularly at the periphery of the tumor, which eventually results in tumor relapse. Chemoembolization can also be administered to the entire liver in several stages, but may accelerate the progression of liver disease. Intrahepatic arterial chemotherapy without embolization may be useful for patients with unresectable hepatocellular carcinoma, particularly with multifocal hepatocellular carcinoma with cirrhosis for which chemoembolization may result in liver failure. By administering chemotherapy into the hepatic artery, the tumor is exposed to the full concentration of the undiluted drug. A number of chemotherapeutic drugs are well tolerated with response rates of up to 40%. Chemotherapy drugs, such as doxorubicin, mitomycin, cisplatin, and fluorouracil, have the added advantage of being metabolized by the liver, which increases their therapeutic ratio by reducing drug concentrations entering the systemic circulation from the liver. Hepatocellular carcinoma is generally poorly responsive to systemic chemotherapy, with response rates of 16% for doxorubicin and 11% for mitomycin. No significant survival benefit has been demonstrated in a small randomized controlled study. Absolute ethanol can be injected percutaneously into hepatic tumors, producing tumor necrosis and survival comparable to chemoembolization. However, the effectiveness of this treatment is limited to tumors <3 cm (<1.2 in) in diameter, probably because of the limitation of the volume of ethanol which can be administered. Liver transplantation can be considered for patients with cirrhosis and heptocellular carcinoma. Results have been best for those with tumors <5 cm (<1.9 in) in diameter.

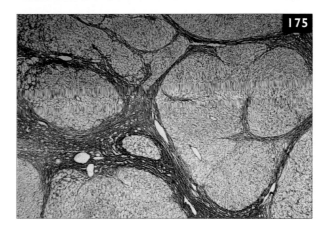

Ascitic fluid:
Protein 5 g/dL (50 g/L)
Albumin 2 g/dL (20 g/L)
LDH 120 U/L
Nucleated cells 200/mm³ (2 × 10⁸/L)
Triglycerides 50 mg/dL (0.56 mmol/L)
Amylase 103 U/L
Negative ascitic fluid cytology

The other investigations show:
Platelet count 114,000/mm³ (114 × 10⁹/L)
Gammaglobulin 1.9 g/dL (19 g/L)
Prothrombin time slightly reduced
Bilirubin 2 mg/dL (34.2 μmol/L)
WBC count 2,400/mm³ (2.4 × 10⁹/L)
Plasma albumin 3.3 g/dL (33 g/L)

175 A 42-year-old alcoholic male presents with a 3 month history of progressively increasing abdominal perimeter. On physical examination a protuberant abdomen with bulging flanks and shifting dullness is noted. An exploratory paracentesis is performed and elicits a yellow fluid. Laboratory investigations are shown.
i. What does the liver biopsy reveal (**175**)?
ii. What is revealed by the analysis of the ascitic fluid?
iii. Should further investigations be undertaken?

175 i. The liver biopsy shows well defined regenerative nodules surrounded by fibrous tracts, diagnostic of liver cirrhosis.

ii. When faced with an ascitic fluid of unknown origin the total protein concentration is the first parameter to consider. The ascites of cirrhotic patients usually shows the characteristics of a transudate, with a total protein concentration of <2.5g/dL (25 g/L). However, these patients do not constitute an homogeneous population, and up to 30% of cirrhotics may exhibit total ascitic protein concentration >3 g/dL (>30 g/L) (exudative ascites). In order to rule out other causes of high protein concentration ascites it is important to calculate the serum–ascites albumin gradient, by substracting the albumin concentration of the ascitic fluid from the albumin concentration of a serum specimen. A gradient of more than 1.1 g/L predicts portal hypertension with great accuracy. This patient has a serum–ascites albumin gradient of 1.3 g/L. Spontaneous bacterial peritonitis can be ruled out because of the absence of a high number of ascitic polymorphonuclear leukocytes. The main conditions that have to be considered in the differential diagnosis are peritoneal carcinomatosis (presenting with high protein concentration and positive ascitic fluid cytology in more than 90% of cases), tuberculous peritonitis (with high protein concentration and increased lymphocyte count), massive liver metastases with portal hypertension, chylous ascites secondary to abdominal lymphoma or trauma, pancreatic ascites (high protein fluid with increased amylase levels), and ascites caused by hepatic venous outflow block.

iii. In order to rule out the conditions mentioned above a number of tests should be undertaken: ascitic fluid levels of amylase, triglycerides, cholesterol; a search for atypical cells in ascitic fluid; a thorough medical history plus Lowenstein cultures to rule out tuberculous peritonitis; hepatic vein catheterization to rule out Budd–Chiari syndrome; ultrasound and CT scan. Laparoscopic examination plus liver biopsy should only be performed when the former investigations do not point to a possible diagnosis.

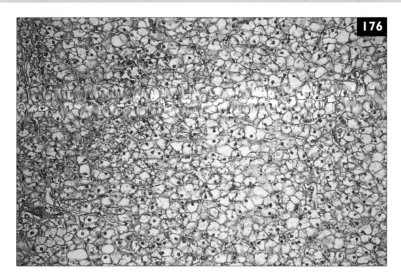

176 A 4-month-old male is brought to the emergency room with a history of a seizure. The past history revealed a normal delivery and neonatal course. The infant is breast fed and just began sleeping through the night. On physical examination, the child is listless and weak. He

Serum glucose 15 mg/dL (0.83 mmol/L)
AST 50 U/L
ALT 47 U/L
Total bilirubin 1.1 mg/dL (18.8 μmol/L)

has a protuberant abdomen and hepatomegaly. Laboratory investigations are shown.
i. Comment on the liver biopsy (H&E) (176).
ii. What is the likely diagnosis?

177 A group of frightened secondary school students present to the emergency room with a friend who felt ill at a party. The patient is a 16-year-old Asian male who experienced palpitations and a flushed 'hot' sensation after drinking two beers. The patient had never consumed alcohol before and he suspected his beer had been poisoned.
i. What is the most likely cause of the young man's discomfort?
ii. Is the reaction experienced by this patient a risk for development of alcoholic liver disease?

176 i. This biopsy demonstrates enlarged hepatocytes with excessive glycogen and fat.
ii. The combination of hepatomegaly with hypoglycemia, only slight elevations in serum transaminase activities, and excessive glycogen on liver biopsy describes glycogen storage disease type I. The glycogen storage diseases are characterized by the accumulation of glycogen in the liver, kidneys, and muscles. Types I, II, III, IV, and VI are associated with liver involvement. Type I usually presents in an infant with hepatomegaly without evidence of hepatocellular dysfunction. Type I is associated with significant hypoglycemia which can result in seizure activity. Platelet dysfunction, and thus bleeding, is also associated with type I. The potential for liver adenoma even in childhood is significant. Hepatic glucose-6-phosphatase is either absent or low. Type II disease is associated with cardiac involvement, and many children die in the first year of life from heart failure. These patients do not develop cholestasis but do present with hepatomegaly. They have a deficiency in lysosomal alpha-1,4-glucosidase. Type III disease is similar to type I. There is a higher incidence of muscle involvement, liver dysfunction with hepatomegaly, and portal fibrosis on liver histology in later childhood. An abnormal glycogen accumulates in the hepatocytes and in other organs. There is a deficiency of amylo-1,6-glucosidase (debrancher enzyme). Type IV disease also has hepatic involvement. Liver histology reveals the accumulation of an abnormal glycogen (amylopectin) in hepatocytes and other organs. There is a deficiency of 1,4 glucan-6-glycosyltransferase (brancher enzyme). Patients typically present at 3–15 months of age with failure to thrive, abdominal distension, hepatosplenomegaly, and jaundice.

Type VI glycogen storage disease is probably the most common form of abnormal glycogen metabolism. There is a deficiency in phosphorylase activity. Patients present with asymptomatic hepatomegaly. There may be growth retardation in infancy.

177 i. The cause of the condition is high circulating catecholamine levels induced by acetaldehyde.
ii. No. The major metabolic pathway of alcohol in human beings is oxidation in the liver. Alcohol is first oxidized to acetaldehyde by ADH in the cytosol of the hepatocyte. Acetaldehyde enters the mitochondria where it is converted to acetate by acetaldehyde dehydrogenase. Acetate is released into the circulation where it is oxidized to fatty acids, carbon dioxide, and water. Acetaldehyde dehydrogenase (ALDH) is the major enzyme that catalyzes the oxidation of acetaldehyde into acetate. There are various forms of hepatic ALDH; ALDH2 codes for ALDH2*1, which is active and ALDH2*2 which is inactive. Lack of activity of this enzyme is believed to result from the substitution of glutamate for lysine. The way alcohol is handled by different individuals is believed to depend on the activity of ALDH.

Some Asians and South American Indians have a predominance of the inactive form of ALDH. Individuals with this deficiency experience an adverse reaction after alcohol ingestion mediated by the release of catecholamines by higher circulating concentrations of acetaldehyde caused by deficiency of ALDH. This unpleasant reaction is characterized by tachycardia, facial flushing, and nausea.

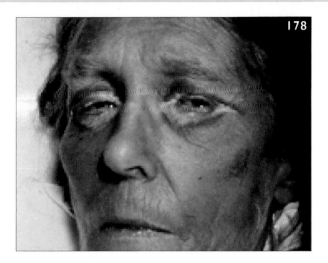

178 A 74-year-old female is referred for evaluation of pruritus of 1 year duration. She has noticed the development of yellow tinged lesions around her eyes and in her ears and palm creases. The lesions are not pruritic. Her appetite is good. Her energy level has been low for the past year. Laboratory investigations are shown.

ALP 433 U/L
ALT 106 U/L
Total bilirubin 1.6 mg/dL (27.36 µmol/L)
IgM 863 mg/dL (8.6 g/L)
Albumin 4.1 g/dL (41 g/L)
Cholesterol 2,217 mg/dL (57.4 mmol/L)

i. What is the most likely diagnosis in this patient?
ii. What are the clinical signs shown (178)?
iii. What is the presumed pathogenesis of this clinical sign?

178 i. Primary biliary cirrhosis is the likely diagnosis.

ii. Cutaneous xanthomata are illustrated.

iii. High serum cholesterol due to cholestasis is associated with xanthomata.

Symptomatic primary biliary cirrhosis typically presents with pruritus, fatigue, and less commonly spontaneous bone fractures in middle-aged women. Biochemical liver tests have a cholestatic pattern. Serum IgM and cholesterol are elevated.

The liver has a central role in lipid metabolism which includes the metabolism of fatty acids, sterols, and lipids classified as complex such as triglycerides, glycerophosphatides, and sphingolipids. The liver also synthesizes numerous proteins that are involved in lipid metabolism including the apolipoproteins, carrier proteins (e.g. albumin, phospholipids, triglycerides, and cholesterol ester), receptors (e.g. ApoB100, ApoB48, ApoE, and albumin) and enzymes (e.g. lecithin cholesterol acyl transferase [LCAT] and hepatic lipase). LCAT plays a major role in the formation of cholesteryl ester from cholesterol in serum.

Fatty acids are taken up by hepatocytes by a receptor-mediated mechanism and are oxidized in the mitochondria and peroxisomes. The liver can continuously uptake fatty acids and export lipoproteins in the form of triglyceride-rich lipoproteins (e.g. VLDL) which contributes to the maintenance of a lipid balance. Another function of the liver is the synthesis of cholesterol. The regulation of body cholesterol by the hepatocyte is unique because cholesterol is excreted in bile and it constitutes the backbone of bile acids. Another function of the liver is the uptake of VLDL by the VLDL receptors expressed on the hepatocyte membrane.

The increase in serum cholesterol in cholestasis is caused primarily by free cholesterol. Studies of lipoprotein metabolism in patients with cholestasis reveal marked elevations of plasma cholesterol and phospholipids. An abnormal LDL known as lipoprotein X (LP-X) was initially described in the plasma of patients with primary biliary cirrhosis. LP-X is rich in phospholipids and free cholesterol, and poor in triglycerides and cholesteryl ester. LP-X can also be found in hepatitis and cirrhosis not of the biliary type.

As cholestasis progresses and liver function decreases so does LCAT activity. This may explain, in part, the accumulation of free cholesterol, lecithin, and LP-X in the plasma of patients with a long history of cholestatic liver disease. As liver failure increases, bile flow decreases markedly, and so does the production of cholesterol and phospholipids. This may account for the low concentration in plasma cholesterol and lecithin in patients with end-stage biliary cirrhosis.

Cutaneous xanthomata are manifestations of the hyperlipidemia that result from cholestasis. They tend to occur around the eyes, in areas of creases (flexor aspect of elbows and hand creases), and areas of pressure and trauma (e.g. elbows and ankles). These lesions are composed primarily of cholesteryl ester. Peripheral neuropathy has been described as a result of lipid deposits on nerves. Dietary restrictions do not resolve the hyperlipidemia of cholestasis. The nonabsorbable resin cholestyramine may reduce the cutaneous xanthomas. Therapy with clofibrate results in a paradoxical increase in serum cholesterol and is not recommended. An increase in coronary artery disease in patients with primary biliary cirrhosis and hyperlipidemia has not been documented.

179 A 60-year-old male presents with a petechial hemorrhage and is found to have a platelet count of 6,000/mm³ (6 × 10⁹/L). A reticulin stain of his bone marrow tissue shows increased reticulin deposition, consistent with the diagnosis of agnogenic myeloid metaplasia (myelofibrosis). He is treated with intravenous methylprednisone and im-

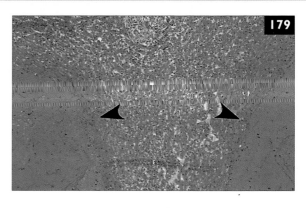

mune globulin and discharged on danazol 100 mg, alternating with 200 mg, daily. He presents with an acute abdomen 1 year later. Examination reveals marked hepatosplenomegaly. A laparotomy is performed which reveals a ruptured spleen with hemoperitoneum and bluish cysts on the hepatic surface. A splenectomy and evacuation of intra-abdominal blood are performed. The postoperative course is complicated by liver failure and he dies on the 10th postoperative day. An autopsy is performed. His liver biopsy results are shown (179).

i. What is revealed in his liver biopsy by the features marked with arrows?
ii. What is the most likely diagnosis?
iii. What is the pathogenesis of this condition?

180 A 24-year-old female presents at the emergency room with unremitting abdominal pain of over 3 hours duration. She describes the sudden onset of right upper quadrant pain that increased in severity and has now plateaued. She

AST 985 U/L
ALT 690 U/L
Bilirubin 6.2 mg/dL (106 μmol/L)
ALP 210 U/L
WBC count 4,200/mm³ (4.2 × 10⁹/L)
WBC differential count 70% neutrophils, 15% lymphocytes, and 15% eosinophils
HBsAg, anti-HBV, IgM anti-HBc, IgM anti-HAV, and anti-HCV absent

has not noticed dark colored urine or passed light colored stools. She has not experienced fevers or chills and is not sexually active. Two weeks previously, her primary care physician prescribed a 10 day course of erythromycin (500 mg four times a day) for treatment of an upper respiratory tract infection. Physical examination is notable for a temperature of 100°F (37.8°C), scleral icterus, right upper quadrant tenderness, and hepatomegaly (14 cm (5.5 in) in breadth in the right midclavicular line). Laboratory investigations are shown. An abdominal ultrasound examination is entirely normal.

i. What is the most likely diagnosis?
ii. What is the pathophysiology of this condition?

179 i. The liver contains large blood-filled cysts (arrows) which have no intact endothelial lining. The features are typical of peliosis hepatis. At this magnification, extramedullary hematopoiesis, a finding that was present secondary to the hematopoietic disorder, cannot be appreciated.

ii. Fatal peliosis of the liver in a patient with agnogenic myeloid metaplasia treated with danazol. The chronological association between the therapy with danazol and the clinicopathological developments suggest a cause and effect relation. The marked replacement of hepatic parenchyma by hematopoietic cells and peliotic cavities probably represents a major factor leading to the development of liver failure post-splenectomy. The hemoperitoneum that preceded the patient's final illness was secondary to splenic rupture from associated splenic peliosis.

iii. The pathogenesis of this disorder is unclear. One hypothesis suggests that peliosis evolves as a result of injury to the sinusoidal endothelium. This theory is supported by several lines of evidence. Ultrastructural studies of the liver from patients with peliosis hepatis demonstrate increased permeability of the endothelial lining of the sinusoidal wall. This results in the passage of RBCs into the space of Disse through enlarged fenestrae. A variety of anabolic and androgenic steroids have been associated with peliosis hepatis. This vascular lesion involving dilation of the sinusoids can appear at any time during anabolic and androgenic steroid treatment and does not depend on the dose used. It is seen in all age groups and is not related to gender. The clinical manifestations include hepatomegaly, tenderness in the right upper quadrant, intraperitoneal hemorrhage following rupture of peliotic lesions, and liver failure secondary to loss of hepatic parenchyma. Frequently, the condition is asymptomatic. Biochemical liver tests are usually normal until the advanced stages of disease. This lesion may regress after cessation of the anabolic and androgenic steroid treatment.

180 i. Erythromycin induced cholestatic hepatitis. The medical history and the laboratory test results strongly suggest drug induced acute hepatocellular disease. Also, the normal ultrasound essentially excludes acute cholecystitis and extrahepatic biliary tract obstruction. The clinical presentation of the lesion can resemble acute cholecystitis or ascending cholangititis so closely that it may not always be possible to distinguish erythromycin hepatotoxicity from biliary tract disease on clinical grounds alone.

ii. The clinical features of fever, eosinophilia, and short latent period between initiation of drug therapy and onset of hepatotoxic manifestations suggest that a hypersensitivity mechanism most likely plays a role. However, erythromycin estolate causes a concentration-dependant impairment of bile flow in the isolated perfused rat liver and inhibition of canalicular membrane Mg^{2+} – and Na^+/K^+-ATPases and a direct hepatotoxic effect of erythromycin may also be involved.

Index

Classification of cases

Q&A Color Reviews feature a question and answer format. Questions are based on cases and illustrated with photographs, diagrams, and x-rays. Answers include discussions on various aspects of the case – differential diagnosis, complications, and management.

Q&A Color Reviews can help you hone your clinical skills, prepare for examinations, and be ready on rounds.

Q&A Color Reviews published in 2003:
Pediatric Emergency Medicine
General Critical Care
Clinical Neurology and Neurosurgery
Hepatobiliary Medicine

The Americas

ISBN 1-58890-152-1

1-58890-152-1 (TNY)

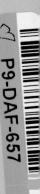

www.thieme.com